Positive Options for

Antiphospholipid Syndrome

Ordering

Trade bookstores in the U.S. and Canada please contact:

Publishers Group West

1700 Fourth Street, Berkeley CA 94710

Phone: (800) 788-3123   Fax: (510) 528-3444

Hunter House books are available at bulk discounts for textbook course adoptions; to qualifying community, health-care, and government organizations; and for special promotions and fund-raising. For details please contact:

Special Sales Department

Hunter House Inc., PO Box 2914, Alameda CA 94501-0914

Phone: (510) 865-5282   Fax: (510) 865-4295

E-mail: sales@hunterhouse.com

Individuals can order our books from most bookstores, by calling **(800) 266-5592**, or from our website at **www.hunterhouse.com**

Positive Options

for

Antiphospholipid Syndrome

Self-Help and Treatment

Triona Holden

Forewords by Graham Hughes, M.D., FRCP
& Robert Roubey, M.D.

Library of Congress Cataloging-in-Publication Data

Holden, Triona.
Positive options for antiphospholipid syndrome : self-help and treatment / Triona Holden; forewords by Graham Hughes and Robert Roubey.— 1st ed,
p. cm.
Includes bibliographical references and index.
ISBN 0-89793-409-1 (pbk.) — ISBN 0-89793-410-5 (cl.)
1. Antiphospholipid syndrome—Popular works. I. Title.
RC600 .H656 2003
616.97'8—dc21   2002152621

Project Credits

Cover Design: Brian Dittmar Graphic Design
Book Production: Hunter House
Copy Editor: Kelley Blewster
Proofreader: John David Marion
Indexer: Nancy D. Peterson
Acquisitions Editor: Jeanne Brondino
Editor: Alexandra Mummery
Publicity Coordinator: Lisa E. Lee
Sales & Marketing Coordinator: Jo Anne Retzlaff
Customer Service Manager: Christina Sverdrup
Order Fulfillment: Lakdhon Lama
Administrator: Theresa Nelson
Computer Support: Peter Eichelberger
Publisher: Kiran S. Rana

Printed and Bound by Bang Printing, Brainerd, Minnesota

Manufactured in the United States of America
9 8 7 6 5 4 3 2 1   First Edition   03 04 05 06 07

Contents

Important Note

The material in this book is intended to provide a review of resources and information related to antiphospholipid syndrome. Every effort has been made to provide accurate and dependable information. However, professionals in the field may have differing opinions, and change is always taking place. Any of the treatments described herein should be undertaken only under the guidance of a licensed health-care practitioner. The author, contributors, editors, publishers, and the experts quoted in the book cannot be held responsible for any error, omission, professional disagreement, outdated material, or adverse outcomes that derive from use of any of the treatments or information resources in this book, either in a program of self-care or under the care of a licensed practitioner.

Foreword to the U.K. Edition

"Listen to the patient, for they are telling you the diagnosis." That was the very first sentence I heard on my introductory ward round as a medical student at the London Hospital. It has stuck with me ever since. I believe it should be the first lesson for every aspiring doctor—and not only for doctors.

In reading the proofs of this book, I was struck by the deft and sympathetic way in which Triona Holden has continued the tradition of listening to the patient. Rarely have I read such a clear and sympathetic approach to a medical condition that is at best complex, at worst daunting. Yet, as Triona Holden points out, antiphospholipid syndrome may come to be the most common and most important of the so-called autoimmune diseases. And it is still underdiagnosed.

Perhaps the simplest way to highlight this fact is to pose the following questions to any doctor with a general practice: Do you have patients with recurrent headache or migraine? Or who have miscarried repeatedly? Or with unexpected thrombosis (blood clotting), for example, deep-vein thrombosis (DVT)? Do you have unexpectedly young patients who suffer memory loss, heart attacks, or stroke? Or with odd neurological problems, perhaps labeled as "atypical multiple sclerosis"? Or with chronic fatigue, aches and pains, and/or depression that don't seem to fit into any clear pattern?

Yes? Of course, there are many possible diagnoses for these problems. But one of them could be antiphospholipid syndrome (APS), also known as Hughes syndrome, or, more colloquially, as "sticky blood"—a condition for which a cheap blood test is available, and for which treatment can change the lives of many, many patients.

In 1983, my colleagues and I published the first of a series of papers describing the syndrome in detail. One of the positive aspects of running large clinics is that, with experience, you begin to spot clinical patterns. Thus it was in my lupus clinic (currently with twenty-five hundred patients on our list) that I noticed a group of people with a distinct clinical set of features. These included thrombosis, neurological disease (especially strokes and headaches, but also movement disorder and memory loss), sometime low platelet counts, livedo reticularis (a blotchy appearance of the skin, in which the veins can be seen through the skin), and the presence in the blood of telltale antibodies called *antiphospholipid antibodies* (APLA).

On every ward round, we doctors would discuss this complex group of patients. As so often happens in medicine, once you spot a clinical picture, the story grows and the number of cases increases—in this case, dramatically.

We pointed out two (I believe) important clinical facts. First, that the condition could affect arteries as well as veins. Second, and crucially, that the condition could occur in the *absence* of lupus, the so-called *primary* antiphospholipid syndrome.

I have gone on record as saying—and I believe this very strongly—that the primary antiphospholipid syndrome will come to be recognized as a more common condition than lupus, and will be shown to bear an impact on conditions as varied as migraine, pregnancy and infertility, neurological problems (including memory loss), and artery disease.

My colleagues and I worked very hard to set up standardized blood tests for APS, and to educate and bring together medical professionals interested in the subject. In 1984, we held the rather grandly named First International Conference on the subject, in London. This was followed in 1986 by the second conference at St. Thomas' Hospital, also in London. Since then, the subject has taken off, with an international conference every two years. The most recent, the ninth, was held in France and attracted eight hundred participants. At the sixth international conference, in Leuven, Belgium, my colleagues honored me by naming the condition *Hughes syndrome* (partly, I suspect, because of the complexity of the more scientific name).

This is an honor I accept with pride. Some eponymous diseases are "small print." In others, the author describes perhaps five or six cases. In this disease, in a series of papers published between 1983 and 1985, we not only described in detail a large number of patients, but filled in much of the clinical picture. The strokes, memory loss, arterial disease, the "primary" syndrome, the pulmonary hypertension, the strong association with recurrent miscarriage, the livedo, the low-platelet tendency, the spinal cord disease—all were carefully documented. But we also developed and standardized anticardiolipin testing, one of the blood tests for APS. Although it would not have been my style to name the syndrome anything other than APS, the "Hughes syndrome" eponym gives me particular pleasure because of the enormous amount of work (ironically, with almost no grant funding) that went into researching and identifying the disorder.

I wish to pay tribute to four colleagues: Dr. Nigel Harris and Aziz Gharavi, who were later joined by Dr. Ron Asherson, each of whom gave his all to the work, and subsequently Dr. Munther Khamashta, who has done so much as my right-hand man to develop research related to the syndrome, especially in the field of recurrent miscarriage.

The syndrome is now established—though it is still insufficiently widely recognized. Cases that in retrospect are shiningly obvious to those of us steeped in clinical practice are still missed. This is why I believe that books such as *Positive Options for Antiphospholipid Syndrome* are so important.

There are few more enjoyable and positive experiences than working with APS patients. Back in 1983, in one of my earliest papers in the *British Medical Journal*, I wrote, "[F]or those of us hardened to nihilism by years of study of various autoantibodies in systemic lupus erythematosus there is a rare sense of excitement at the implications of the associations now being reported."

The same holds true today.

— Graham Hughes, M.D., FRCP
Head of the Lupus Research Unit at St. Thomas' Hospital, London

Foreword to the U.S. Edition

I am delighted to write a forward for the US edition of this important and timely book on the Antiphospholipid Syndrome (APS). Triona Holden's courageous story of her own illness and the moving stories of other patients with APS will certainly increase awareness of the syndrome and offer much needed information and comfort to many.

Fortunately, awareness of APS in the medical community is growing. As the cases in this book demonstrate, the various manifestations of APS involve multiple medical specialties—rheumatology, hematology, neurology, obstetrics, and dermatology. Nearly all of the specialists in these fields are now aware of the syndrome and its most common features (blood clots in arteries and veins and miscarriages). General internists and family doctors are becoming more interested and knowledgeable about APS, although more education is needed. Some of the features that figure prominently in many of the cases described by Ms. Holden, particularly chronic headache, difficulty with thinking, and multiple sclerosis-like symptoms, are less well known, however. This is due, in large part, to the genuine need for more research in these areas.

Patients and their families should take heart in the fact that APS research efforts are growing and yielding important new information. One or more sessions devoted to APS research are now regularly included in national and international rheumatology and coagulation meetings. Further, the international symposia devoted exclusively to APS, currently held every two years, continue to expand. The most recent symposium, the tenth, was held in Sicily in the fall of 2002. It lasted five days and was attended by approximately six hundred physicians and scientists from around the world. It also included an international consensus workshop on APS treatment.

I would like to add a few comments that may assist readers in understanding APS and the cases presented by Ms. Holden. The terminology surrounding APS can be confusing to patients and their families. The adjectives "thick" and "thin" as they apply to blood should be clarified. These words describe conditions in which the blood clots more easily than normal (thick) or less easily than normal (thin). In the context of APS when we say that the blood is too thick, we mean that there is a greater than normal tendency for blood clots to form. It does not mean that the blood is actually thicker or more viscous. Similarly, when we talk about "blood thinners" we mean medications that cause blood to clot less readily than normal. "Blood thinners" do not actually make blood more watery or less viscous. "Sticky blood" is another term meaning that the blood clots more readily than normal. The blood itself is not actually sticky, in the common sense of that word, although in some blood clotting diseases certain blood cells, such as platelets, may tend to clump together or stick to blood vessel walls. "Sticky blood" is certainly a very useful way to describe the increased risk of blood clotting in APS, although it is not a specific term for this disease. APS, although it has unique features, is only one of many conditions in which blood clots too readily. Indeed, it is important for patients with blood clots and/or miscarriages who are being tested for APS to also have a thorough evaluation for other causes of "sticky blood."

Another area of confusion for patients and their families involves the laboratory tests for antiphospholipid antibodies. Most experts in the field recommend testing for anticardiolipin antibodies and lupus anticoagulants, as described in the book. Unfortunately, test results may sometimes vary from laboratory to laboratory (despite considerable improvements in test standardization in recent years). Most often this occurs with samples that fall near the borderline between negative and low positive values. Repeat testing over time and assessment by a physician with experience diagnosing APS may be helpful.

Some commercial laboratories offer large panels of antiphospholipid antibody tests, similar to anticardiolipin tests, but using other phospholipids (phosphatidylserine, phosphatidylinositol, phosphatidic acid, etc.). In general, these tests are not standardized, and the significance of one of these tests being positive (if routine anticardiolipin and lupus anticoagulant tests are negative) is not known. Further, these tests may be quite expensive. At the present time most experts in the field do not recommend testing for antibodies to a panel of different phospholipids.

As a result of exciting research in the field, new laboratory tests for APS are emerging. There is strong evidence that most of the antibodies detected in anticardiolipin tests and some of the antibodies detected in lupus anticoagulant tests do not actually target phospholipids, but rather a protein in the blood called β_2-glycoprotein I. Other lupus anticoagulant antibodies appear to be directed against another blood protein, prothrombin. Tests for antibodies to β_2-glycoprotein I are available and, in certain situations, may offer some advantages over anticardiolipin and lupus anticoagulant tests. Tests for antibodies to prothrombin are also available, although their role is the diagnosis of APS is not yet clear. A full explanation of these newer tests and the situations in which they may be helpful is beyond the scope of this forward, but it is an area some patients may wish to discuss with their doctors.

The diagnosis of APS is sometimes difficult, even for physicians with experience treating the condition. There remain a number of patients with problems very suggestive of APS who are consistently negative in antiphospholipid tests done by reputable laboratories. Speculatively, some of these patients might have autoantibodies similar to antiphospholipid antibodies, but that are not detected in currently available laboratory tests. Others may have conditions unrelated to APS. While this is a promising area for research, it may be a difficult situation for patients and their doctors.

Lastly, I would like to add a few words about Dr. Graham Hughes, who figures prominently in Ms. Holden's book. Graham has been a valued teacher, colleague, and friend for nearly twenty years. In the mid 1980s, during my postdoctoral training, I had the opportunity to spend about six months in London working with Graham and his group. This was a busy and exciting time as the full picture of APS was just emerging. Beyond Graham's contributions to APS research and experience in treating patients, one thing that comes through clearly in this book is his ability and willingness to listen carefully to patients. I witnessed this on a regular basis during my time in England, and have tried to emulate it in my career. Not only is listening carefully to patients essential for excellent medical care, it is also crucial for research. One thing that may not be evident from the book is Graham's extraordinary ability to see patterns and connections among patients and to generate new and creative ideas for laboratory research. This is a rare and special talent, and one that has greatly benefited Graham's many students and trainees, and all patients suffering from APS.

— Robert A. S. Roubey, M.D.
    Director, Antiphospholipid Syndrome Collaborative Registry
        (APSCORE)
    Associate Professor of Medicine
    Division of Rheumatology & Immunology
    University of North Carolina at Chapel Hill
    May 2003

Introduction

I was working on an article for *The London Times* when I first stumbled across the condition known as "sticky blood." The piece I was writing was about lupus, a topic that interested me because I suffer from the illness. I had been interviewing one of the world's leading specialists in lupus, Dr. Graham Hughes. We were huddled in his office at St. Thomas' Hospital in Central London, and I'd been grilling him for an hour or so. Things were going well, as he is a consummate performer in front of journalists and had given me plenty of strong quotes. The interview was winding down and I was about to shove my notebook back into my bag when Dr. Hughes began talking about antiphospholipid syndrome (APS). I must have looked dumbstruck by this mouthful because he quickly explained that it was a relatively new condition known in lay terms as "sticky blood," and that it would eventually be identified as the most common autoimmune disease of this century.

Instinctively I picked up my notebook again and began to scribble. After twenty years as a journalist you develop a nose for what we call a "cracking tale," and this sounded like just that.

With the calm of a man talking about the weather, Dr. Hughes described the syndrome that thickened the blood and thereby caused clots. It affected men and women, young and old alike. It attacked any part of the body at any time. Sticky blood was responsible for a quarter of recurrent miscarriages and a fifth of strokes in young people. It was often mistaken for multiple sclerosis (MS) or early Alzheimer's. It caused deep-vein thrombosis, including so-called economy-class syndrome, memory loss, speech difficulties, headaches, fatigue, and joint pains. It damaged major organs and caused blindness or even death.

Another key concern was the fact that many patients struggled for years to get a diagnosis and were often misdiagnosed, mainly as a result of medical ignorance about the syndrome. Recently at one clinic three people who'd been told they had MS were tested and then advised that in fact they had APS (also known as Hughes syndrome). The difference between the two illnesses could not be more profound. MS consigns the sufferer to what can be an appalling degenerative condition. It manifests in varying degrees of severity, but no matter how it affects someone, the treatments available for the symptoms are limited and very expensive. By contrast, a broad range of medications have been shown to be highly effective in the treatment of APS. These drugs are generally inexpensive and easily available; aspirin is one example.

That was the good news about antiphospholipid syndrome, the "magic," as Dr. Hughes would say. It was highly treatable with medication that thinned the blood; even something as mild as children's aspirin could work. The cost of treatment was minimal, and there was an excellent chance that with the right monitoring a patient would live a normal life. The moving stories of the people who suffer from APS that are presented in this book bear that out, such as the one about the woman who was virtually blind and after a few weeks of treatment got her eyesight back, or the former British Airways flight attendant who found herself confined to a wheelchair, unable to control fierce spasms in her lower body. After one week of treatment she was walking with the aid of crutches and is now striding up and down hospital corridors helping others who suffer from APS by tirelessly devoting her time to the Hughes Syndrome Foundation.

Dr. Hughes said that the area where the greatest triumphs against this disease have come is in the fight against complications in pregnancy. Women who had suffered through the agony of repeated miscarriages, including one woman who had had a shocking twenty miscarriages, were given anticoagulants and had gone on to have healthy babies. The pictures that cling to the walls of Dr. Hughes' office are mainly of mothers and children with beaming smiles. After Hughes' team refined the treatment protocol for APS, the pregnancy clinic showed a success rate that rose from under 20 percent to over 75 percent.

I am not known for being lost for words, but there was a moment when my mouth fell open and I was silent. The weight of what I had heard was staggering. Here we had a new condition that was common but as yet seriously underdiagnosed. It touched on several areas of medicine and affected a significant slice of the population, not just in Britain, where it was first identified, but all over the world. A plethora of questions came to mind; the most pressing was why hadn't I heard of Hughes syndrome?

One reason could be that it is still a "new" disease, first identified by Dr. Hughes in the early 1980s. Another issue is the age-old problem of funding. To conduct extensive research or to employ the staff and time required to get the message out takes money, a commodity that is not in large supply in this field of medicine. Those involved in treating patients are too busy doing just that and can't spend their days worrying about publicity. Rather like the case with HIV or lupus, it takes time for the medical community and general public to recognize new conditions.

As a sufferer of lupus, I know firsthand how difficult it is to cope with having an autoimmune disease for which the range of symptoms is broad and diverse. The biggest hurdle is the first: actually getting the diagnosis. When I became ill, but before I had a name for my condition, there were so many things wrong with me that I wrestled with the fear I was going mad. I tried to ignore my symptoms for as long as I could, hoping they would go away— not an easy task when I could no longer pick up my children for a cuddle without experiencing excruciating pain in my shoulders and chest, and muscle weakness in my arms. Worst of all was the fatigue. For someone who relied on having a lot of energy, waking up to a dead battery was as good as a prison sentence. It took two years and a plethora of tests to get a diagnosis. I felt like a laboratory animal, but I appreciated any efforts made to give my illness a name. It sounds odd, but when my condition was diagnosed as a form of systemic lupus erythematosus (SLE), I actually felt delighted—not because I was told I had an incurable and potentially life-threatening disease, but because at long last I had a name for my condition. Having one meant I could find out more about the illness and fight it.

As is the case with lupus, getting a diagnosis for antiphospholipid syndrome is notoriously difficult. The campaign to improve awareness of lupus has been hard fought for over a decade. By contrast, APS is still virtually under wraps. This means that so far only limited information is available to the public. A trawl through bookshops will likely leave you empty-handed. A search on the Internet will yield some websites that are helpful; that of the Hughes Syndrome Foundation is one (www.hughes-syndrome.org). From it you can order a book written by Dr. Hughes, titled *Hughes Syndrome: A Patient's Guide*, which gives an excellent explanation of the disease from a medical perspective.

But if you are like me, you always want more. You want to hear from fellow sufferers so you can compare notes. That is why *Positive Options for Antiphospholipid Syndrome: Self-Help and Treatment* is built around a core of people who have APS and are happy to tell their stories. Perhaps reading about what they went through will prompt others to put the pieces of the puzzle together, bringing them one step closer to getting some answers and stopping this disease from doing any more damage. Chapters 2 through 9 each addresses a specific health problem caused by APS—from blood clotting to miscarriage, strokes to headache. It is in the patients' stories featured in those chapters that you will read in detail about how APS manifests itself in the symptoms of these various health ailments. But first, Chapter 1 offers basic information about the disease. Chapter 10 discusses the often frustrating fight to get a diagnosis of APS in the face of lack of awareness about it in the medical community; Chapter 11 covers an emergency manifestation of the disorder, called *catastrophic antiphospholipid syndrome*; and Chapter 12 goes into greater detail about tests for and treatment of APS.

After hearing about sticky blood from Dr. Hughes, I wrote an article for *The London Times* that triggered a staggering response from readers. They jammed the switchboard at St. Thomas' Hospital and generated more than seventy thousand hits on the Hughes Syndrome Foundation website in a matter of days. I couldn't help but feel that I was just scratching the surface and that there was a pressing need to make more information available to the public at large. Hence this book.

When you find you have a major illness, you unwillingly and unwittingly join a club. Only fellow members can understand the dreadful reality of what you are going through. As a fully paid-up member of the "chronic-illness club," I feel qualified to know something of what it is you need. I am a journalist, not a doctor, so I approach the subject from the point of view of the layperson. I have tried to plow through the medical jargon, sift out the facts, and present them to you so that they can be easily understood. It is important to remember that you are not alone; that is why so many APS patients have happily agreed to talk openly in this book about what happened to them. As "club members," they know how lonely and depressing illness can be.

As a news correspondent who has traveled widely, I have met many remarkable people, and Dr. Graham Hughes is one of them. His dedication to his patients makes him stand out among medical professionals. One thing I have come across time and time again in the people he has treated is that they hold him in the highest esteem. I believe it is right that a remarkable person gets the kind of recognition he or she deserves. Dr. Hughes is the only living doctor in the world to have a disease named after him. Unfortunately, there is some confusion on a global level about the name of the disease. In the United States it has become known as antiphospholipid syndrome and as Hughes syndrome. Here in Britain it has a third name—"sticky blood." I deal in more detail with this issue in Chapter 1, but from my perspective, I think credit should go to where it is due, in this case to Dr. Hughes.

Antiphospholipid syndrome is fairly common; however, in terms of its recognition in the medical community and in the public at large, it is still in its early days, so you will have to do more research than those who will follow in your footsteps. It is crucial that you hang onto the knowledge that there is plenty you can do about this disease if you test positive for it. The key is to get the diagnosis. To do that, you need to know what to look for, whom to insist on seeing, and what tests and treatment you might require. The stance I take in this book is that a proactive patient—one who isn't content merely to sit back and accept without question what she or he is told by medical professionals—is the equivalent to the proverbial squeaky wheel that gets the grease. I hope *Positive Options for Antiphospholipid Syndrome* gives you the information, support, and encouragement you need to become a proactive patient and to fight the good fight.

— Triona Holden, 2003

Chapter 1

Know the Enemy

In a war, one of the most effective weapons you can have is intelligence. It is vital to gain as much information about the enemy as possible. The same scenario applies to any illness, and it is particularly true with antiphospholipid syndrome. Although in the next decade most people will have heard of this condition, at the moment it is relatively new, and awareness of it is frustratingly limited among the general public and, worse, within the medical profession. It is therefore wise to arm yourself with as much information as you can; by doing so, you improve your chances of getting yourself seen by the right experts and of receiving the treatment that could be lifesaving. It is also possible that you will end up knowing more than some of the medical professionals who examine you.

Basics about the Disease

First things first. Let's tackle the name of the condition. Its scientific name is *antiphospholipid syndrome* (abbreviated as *APS* or *APLS*), and this is the name by which it is still most commonly identified in many areas of the world, including the United States. Some medical professionals in the United States use the term *antiphospholipid antibody syndrome*, or *APLA syndrome*. I know these names are a mouthful, and they probably mean nothing at all to you unless you are medically trained. I will go into what they mean later.

In the United Kingdom, the condition is more widely referred to as *Hughes syndrome*, in honor of the renowned British physician Dr. Graham Hughes, who first identified it. Another name for it is *sticky blood*, a term that was coined by the media. The term is not scientific, nor is it completely accurate, but it cleverly describes what the condition actually does. It is also easier to remember and to spell than the word *antiphospholipid*! In this book I use all these names interchangeably, but since I am British, and in keeping with my British-based research about the illness, I most often use the name *Hughes syndrome*.

The next step is to get an idea of what the disease is and how it works. The battleground is within your own body. The enemy is the very mechanism that would normally protect you, namely your immune system. Hughes syndrome is diverse and fickle; it is a condition that recognizes few medical boundaries. This is because of how it works. In simple terms, the immune system turns against itself and becomes overactive. (Read more about how the immune system malfunctions in Hughes syndrome later in this chapter.) The body is fighting imaginary intruders, and as a result the blood becomes thicker and is therefore more likely to clot. Because blood flows through every part of the body, the disease has free access to wherever it decides to target. It can strike anyone, regardless of sex or age. Those affected range from toddlers suffering strokes to seniors having blood clots. It can affect any part of the body at any time for no apparent reason. There is no limit to the range of the disease; sufferers can endure mild symptoms and live a relatively normal life, or they can be so ill they are confined to a bed or wheelchair. In the worst cases, Hughes syndrome can be fatal.

The disease can mimic other illnesses, a fact that makes it difficult to diagnose. Doctors specializing in this field are finding a significant number of patients being referred to them who have been told they are probably in the early stages of multiple sclerosis. Then when they are given the simple blood test for APS, it comes back positive. The difference between MS and Hughes syndrome could not be more profound. MS can be a progressively and permanently debilitating disease, whereas the symptoms of Hughes syndrome are highly treatable and can be effectively controlled. Chapter 6 in this book deals with the differences between MS and Hughes syndrome.

Besides the challenges imposed by the fact that this disorder mimics other illnesses, getting a diagnosis of Hughes syndrome is also difficult because of the variety of symptoms it presents. Moreover, doctors won't find Hughes syndrome if they are not looking for it. Anyone who has been suffering from an unidentified cluster of symptoms for months or possibly years dreads seeing their doctor and hearing yet again, "I'm afraid we just don't know." Those few words can be devastating if you are the one feeling awful. You begin to wonder whether you have been imagining all those ailments; you worry that perhaps you are behaving like a hypochondriac. I have interviewed many APS sufferers who had been told that they were having a hysterical reaction and for whom antidepressants were dished out. Hopefully, reading this book will help convince some people that they are not losing their marbles; they are just unwell.

Hughes syndrome is not really a rare condition, but it may seem to be because so few people have heard of it. In Britain, it is estimated to be responsible for a quarter of all recurrent miscarriages and for one in five strokes in people under age forty. In the United States, antiphospholipid antibodies (APLA) have been reported present in 11–22 percent of women who have had recurrent miscarriages. The word about APS is getting out as more information becomes available. Dr. Hughes is quite clear on the question of how common it is. He states, "I believe that this syndrome will become the most diagnosed autoimmune disease of the twenty-first century—more prevalent than rheumatoid arthritis, lupus, MS, or ME [myalgic encephalomyelitis, better known as chronic fatigue syndrome]." It is possible that as many as one in two hundred people in high-risk groups would prove positive for

Hughes syndrome. Considered worldwide, that is a staggering number.

If you are reading this book, it means you have most likely heard of APS, sticky blood, or Hughes syndrome. It also means you suspect or know that you or someone close to you has the condition. You have probably been desperately searching for more information and have found that precious little is available at the moment. This book aims to provide answers to your questions. In addition, the Resources section, at the back of the book, will direct you to other sources of information.

Signs and Symptoms

What should you look for if you suspect that you have Hughes syndrome? Each patient is different, but a number of danger signs exist, including:

- Any blood clots (thrombosis) in either the veins or arteries;

- Recurrent miscarriage. Doctors regard this as meaning three or more miscarriages, but Graham Hughes thinks tests should be done after even one miscarriage that occurs late-term;

- Strokes, especially in people under forty years of age;

- Memory loss, speech difficulties, symptoms of early Alzheimer's;

- Headaches, migraines, and seizures;

- Pins and needles, trouble balancing or seeing, symptoms associated with multiple sclerosis;

- Extreme fatigue;

- Muscle pains and cramping;

- ◆ Blotchy skin, known by doctors as *livedo reticularis*, in which the blood vessels can be seen under the skin;

- ◆ Low platelet count, which can lead to bruising.

Testing for APS

If a doctor suspects you might have Hughes syndrome, two simple, inexpensive, and conclusive blood tests are available worldwide. The first test is for *anticardiolipin antibodies*, commonly referred to as *a*CL or sometimes ACLA. The second test is for a substance with a confusing name, *lupus anticoagulant*, or LA—confusing because it is not a test for lupus. (More about these tests is covered in Chapter 12.) The science behind these tests is that normally the body has its own natural protection against too much clotting, but in a patient with Hughes syndrome, the immune system produces antibodies that make the blood far more "sticky" and therefore more likely to clot. These antibodies alter the shape of the platelets and the walls of the blood vessels, conditions that in turn affect the free blow of blood.

Antibodies are proteins manufactured by specialized white blood cells. Another name for them is *immunoglobulins*. They are an important part of the immune system, the body's method of resisting disease. Antibodies work by attacking substances that the body recognizes as foreign. Viruses and some bacteria are examples of foreign substances acted upon by antibodies. However, as alluded to earlier in the chapter, sometimes the immune system malfunctions, misinterprets the body's own tissues as foreign, and sends specialized antibodies called *autoantibodies* to attack those tissues, resulting in an *autoimmune reaction*. Antiphospholipid syndrome is an autoimmune disease. (Other examples of autoimmune diseases include lupus, multiple sclerosis, insulin-dependent diabetes, rheumatoid arthritis, and some forms of thyroid illness.) In Hughes syndrome, the body misidentifies phospholipids (a type of fat molecule that forms part of every normal cell's membrane) as foreign and produces antibodies against them. There are several types of antiphospholipid antibodies, but establishing the presence in the blood of the two listed above, LA and aCL, has been established by medical experts as the best way of determining that someone has APS.

Originally, it was thought that only individuals with lupus (systemic lupus erythematosus, or SLE) carried the antiphospholipid antibodies. Then Dr. Hughes and his team determined that people could have APS independently of lupus. APS that occurs by itself is sometimes called *primary APS* (or *primary Hughes syndrome*); when it accompanies lupus or a related disease, it is called *secondary APS* (or *secondary Hughes syndrome*). (Read more about the link between lupus and APS in Chapter 9.)

Possible Causes

What causes Hughes syndrome? At the moment no one knows why the body begins manufacturing antiphospholipid antibodies. Some evidence indicates that there could be a genetic link, and some of the patients whose stories are told in this book feel certain that the condition has run in their families undetected for generations. Autoimmune conditions do tend to run in families. It is frustrating to be unable to point to a cause and say, "There, that's the culprit," but as with many autoimmune conditions, things just aren't that straightforward. That said, you might want to quiz members of your family or check your family history to see if older generations suffered from thrombosis, strokes, recurrent miscarriages, severe headaches, or even growing pains. It is possible that the clues you need to trace your illness are staring out at you from the family tree.

People often ask if the illness has to do with stress. There is no simple answer to that question. Dr. Hughes has found that a link does seem to exist, but no research has yet backed this up. From my conversations with patients, it is quite clear that they often believe a direct connection exists between a major event in their lives and a flare-up of the disease. Some find that even when they are on medication for APS, an increase in stress, such as losing a job or the breakup of a marriage, will act as a trigger for the symptoms to return. It makes sense that a terrible event in someone's life will affect his or her health, especially if that health is already erratic.

Evidence also exists that a viral infection might trigger sticky blood. Patients have reported first noticing a sore throat or a case of the flu, just before beginning to suffer from the symptoms of Hughes syndrome. Is diet a factor? No one knows. The current wisdom for Hughes syndrome is the same as it is for virtually any illness: Eat a balanced diet and get regular exercise. There is no evidence that following such advice works to ameliorate the symptoms, but there is no evidence that it doesn't.

Basics about Treatment

Some APS patients turn to alternative medicines, but the effectiveness of these medicines is tricky to judge. The mainstream treatment is hard to beat, and there is plenty of evidence that it works and can improve symptoms within days if not hours, often without nasty side effects.

What is the most commonly prescribed treatment for Hughes syndrome? It is the use of drugs to thin the blood. Think of it logically: If you have thick blood, the answer must be to thin it. It sounds so simple, and in a way it is. The pharmaceutical industry has developed a whole range of drugs known as *anticoagulants*. These include warfarin (often referred to by its brand name, Coumadin), heparin, and, most common of all, aspirin. Side effects can occur with each of these drugs, but the incidence of such effects varies with the individual. New versions of the drugs are being developed all the time. (Read more about these three medications in Chapter 12.)

Monitoring

Once a patient is diagnosed as having Hughes syndrome, it is imperative that his or her blood be monitored. Doctors keep a close eye on the *INR*, or *internationally normalized ratio*, a set of numbers for determining whether the blood falls within the range for what is regarded as a normal blood thickness. The test to check INR is most often carried out in a doctor's office, hospital, or lab, although home test kits are available. Even a tiny fluctuation in the INR can result in the return of such symptoms as slurred speech, headaches, vision disturbance, blood clots, and mini-strokes. Many patients who have lived with their condition for years have become such experts at recognizing the warning signs that they get help before they become extremely ill yet again.

Migraine, "Multiple Sclerosis," and Memory Loss

by Graham Hughes, M.D., FRCP

Triona Holden asked me to contribute some material on the neurological aspects of antiphospholipid syndrome (APS, also known as Hughes syndrome). I am more than pleased to do so, for I believe that this aspect of the disease will someday come to be recognized as one of the most important.

The successful treatment of women who suffer from APS-related miscarriages has grabbed the headlines—and quite rightly so. Rarely can there be a more clear and satisfying outcome than a successful pregnancy in a woman with previous miscarriages who has been treated for APS. However, there are many other features of the disease, which is a blood-clotting disorder that can affect any organ of the body. One such organ is the brain. For some reason, the brain is peculiarly susceptible to the "sludging," or clotting, of the blood seen in APS—and when the brain is starved of oxygen, the responses are fairly predictable. Three of those responses are headache, a cluster of symptoms often incorrectly identified as multiple sclerosis, and memory loss.

Headache and Migraine

When we at the Hughes Syndrome Foundation set up our patient-advice website (www.hughes-syndrome.org), we received over twenty thousand hits in the first week. Far and away the most common symptom complaint was headache. Many patients with APS give a history of "teenage migraine," sometimes severe, with nausea and flashing lights. Oddly, this headache tendency often disappears, only to return with a vengeance.

Many types of headache exist, and all varieties are capable of happening in APS. The presence of severe, daily headache is a very important clue to the diagnosis.

"Multiple Sclerosis" Symptoms

Another way in which a compromised nervous system can complain is with pins and needles, speech disturbance, giddiness, vertigo, and even leg paralysis—all symptoms of multiple sclerosis. Not surprisingly, a number of patients with APS are initially suspected of having multiple sclerosis. I believe that the number of patients with APS who have incorrectly received a diagnosis of MS is probably far higher than what is currently thought.

And yet the treatment for APS is totally different from that for MS. In the series of patients about whom we recently published articles in the medical literature, an interesting observation was made: When the correct diagnosis of APS was made and anticoagulant treatment started, in all but two patients there was a complete halt in the progression of the neurological disease.

Memory Loss

I personally think that the biggest story of all, as far as this syndrome is concerned, is memory loss. Because the patient isn't asked about it, the history may not come out. Asked about memory loss, however, and the story is dramatic; people describe "memory like a sieve," or being "the joke of the family," or they'll say, "I thought I was developing Alzheimer's," or, "I kept coming out with completely the wrong word"—all, in various ways, features of many APS patients.

I am sure that over the next few years we will see many medical articles about this aspect of the disease, especially since the improvement, once treatment is started, can be so dramatic.

Treatment

At present one or another method of "thinning" the blood—with aspirin, heparin, or warfarin (Coumadin)—is the standard treatment. In many patients, one "junior" or "baby" aspirin (75–100 milligrams) per day is all it takes. The headaches disappear and the memory improves. Even the "multiple sclerosis" features can get better. In others, aspirin is not enough. The medical judgement as to whether to try warfarin is often a major decision. As a compromise, we have suggested a two-week trial of heparin, self-administered by the patient, to assess response.

Ultimately, most patients with major features of Hughes syndrome end up on warfarin, sometimes with the most striking results. The memory improves—"like a fog lifting"—the speech disturbance disappears, the giddiness often vanishes, and the headaches stop. Conversely, when the treatment with anticoagulation falls below the required level and the blood "thickens up" again, the headaches and memory loss return.

One of the most considered lessons we have learned about our patients who show the neurological features of Hughes syndrome is that the patient "knows" when his or her treatment level is right—perhaps an argument in some patients for self-testing anticoagulation kits.

One still wonders how many patients (or their relatives) are out there attending migraine clinics or struggling under the wrong label of "Alzheimer's" or "MS." And yet they are so treatable.

How Can You Help Yourself?

The best way a person with APS can help himself or herself is by getting the proper diagnosis and treatment. Yet doing so can be a challenge, because one of the major problems with the illness at this stage is the lack of awareness about it among medical professionals. That's why it is vital for Hughes syndrome patients to be proactive.

What do I mean by "proactive"? I mean you must be the kind of patient who informs yourself about the illness and your treatment options rather than merely waiting for your doctor to tell you what to do. I will repeat some advice included in another book on a different health-related topic: It says, in essence, if you wish to simply follow your doctor's instructions without question and go blindly into treatment, or if you wish to bury your head in the sand

and do little or nothing to help yourself, then this book isn't for you. If, however, you want to learn everything you can about the disease and about what to expect, then keep reading. Such a person wants to take an active role in his or her health care. Such a person wants to do everything possible to survive and thrive. Research has shown that patients with life-threatening illnesses who take an active role in their health care live longer and enjoy a better quality of life than those who don't. To help yourself in the battle against Hughes syndrome, then, you must start by deciding to do so.

The following are some ideas you can use if you want to be a proactive patient:[1]

- ◆ Many APS sufferers end up seeing several doctors and specialists before getting the proper diagnosis and treatment. Some Hughes syndrome patients believe that the best way to get in front of the right doctor is through a clinic affiliated with a university medical school. When calling to make an appointment, ask if the school has any specialists knowledgeable about antiphospholipid syndrome. You might also try asking to see a specialist in autoimmune disorders.

- ◆ Because Hughes syndrome can be linked with lupus (SLE), sometimes a doctor specializing in lupus will also be knowledgeable about Hughes syndrome. Make an appointment with a lupus clinic. If there isn't one in your area, make an appointment with a rheumatologist (a doctor who specializes in treating, among other things, certain autoimmune disorders). To find a rheumatologist in your area, visit the website of the American College of Rheumatology (see Resources).

- ◆ Some APS patients have had success working with hematologists (doctors specializing in the blood). To find a hematologist, start with your local yellow pages, where doctors are listed under their specialties.

◆ Get a referral from another APS patient. How do you find other patients with this disease? Several excellent online support groups exist for antiphospholipid syndrome (see Resources). Post a message asking if anyone can recommend a good doctor near where you live.

◆ Once you've made a doctor's appointment, prepare for it. Make a list of questions to ask the doctor, based on what you've read in this book and what you've learned from your online discussion group. Leave space to write the answers.

◆ Make sure the doctor has the relevant information about your health before you show up for your appointment. This includes test results, changes in your symptoms, and other doctors' assessments of your condition. Work with your current doctor to get your chart sent to the new doctor. You should also consider typing up a list of your symptoms—along with the approximate dates of their onset—and faxing or mailing it the new doctor before your first appointment.

◆ Take someone with you to your doctor appointments. Ask the person to take notes during the visit. Another person may be able to ask clearer and tougher questions than you can. At the very least, you will have two sets of ears listening to what the doctor says. If you are single, or if your spouse or partner is too emotional about your health problems, take a trusted friend or family member.

◆ Your doctor may use technical terms and introduce complicated concepts. Ask him or her to stop and explain these. If the doctor's explanation doesn't make sense to you, ask him or her to clarify the issue again, perhaps in a different way.

◆ Make sure that you thoroughly understand any tests and/or treatments prescribed by your doctor. Ask detailed questions about their purpose, necessity, and possible side effects.

◆ Continue keeping a log of your symptoms. Include a description of each one and the dates that it flared up and subsided. Take the list to every doctor appointment.

◆ Some patients with chronic illness believe that it pays to insist on obtaining copies of all test results and X rays, rather than simply accepting without question what the doctor or lab tells them. They have found that mistakes occur too often in lab work and in the transfer of information back and forth between medical professionals. They maintain that it is worth educating themselves to be able to read and interpret their own lab results. Your test results and all communications about you between health professionals belong to you by law; obtaining copies of them will require asserting yourself, but doing so may be worth it.

◆ Even though you may already have seen several doctors and may be tired of visiting new specialists, don't be afraid to change doctors if you don't like one. Pay special attention to whether or not a doctor seems respectful of your desire for information. As one pamphlet for APS patients puts it, a doctor who doesn't want informed patients isn't the right doctor for you. Keep looking until you find a doctor who will work *with* you to manage your care.

Now that we have gathered some basic intelligence about antiphospholipid syndrome, and have discussed the necessity of taking an active role in your own treatment, let's look in more detail at the different ways the disorder can affect people. The next several chapters are each devoted to discussing a specific health problem caused by the illness. In them, you will meet APS patients who, once they and their doctors established the right diagnosis and determined the right treatment, enjoyed improved health—sometimes drastically so. Even if a chapter is about a symptom of Hughes syndrome that hasn't affected you, it will still benefit you to read the chapter, because many of the principles of managing the illness are the same no matter whether the patient's primary symptom is blood clots, recurrent miscarriage, or neurological problems. General conclusions can also be drawn from the case studies included at the end of most chapters.

It is my hope that these individuals' stories will encourage and inform you about the positive options available to you for dealing with APS.

Chapter 2

Blood Clots

Have you ever had a clot in a blood vessel, technically called a *thrombus*? It doesn't matter where, when, or how serious it was. What matters is whether you have suffered at all from thrombosis (the condition of having a thrombus). If the answer is yes, then it is possible you have Hughes syndrome—that your blood contains the antiphospholipid antibodies that make it thicker than it ought to be. This condition puts you at risk of having additional, possibly more serious, clots. You should insist on getting the blood tests that will determine whether you have antiphospholipid syndrome. (More information about these tests is provided in Chapter 12.)

The Dangers Posed by Clotting

The areas most commonly affected by clots are the veins in the legs and arms, but clots can also affect smaller veins in organs such as the kidney, liver, and eyes. One of the greatest dangers with a clot is that it might break up and travel to another part of the body, such as the heart, brain, or lungs. In any of these vital areas a clot can prove fatal. Before this happens, patients may suffer minor clots, which are regarded as early warnings.

Another aspect of clotting in Hughes syndrome is that, unlike other clotting disorders, it can cause thrombosis in the arteries as well as in the veins. A clot in an artery, which will affect major organs like the brain and the heart, has much more severe consequences than one in a vein. An arterial clot can cause what is known as a *TIA* (transient ischemic attack) in the brain; this can lead to permanent memory loss, speech difficulties, headaches, seizures, and strokes. A thrombus in an artery can also lead to angina or heart attack.

The presence of a blood clot is the singular most dramatic sign that someone might be suffering from APS.

Deep-Vein Thrombosis and APS

A lot has been written in recent years about deep-vein thrombosis, or DVT. The legs contain two major groups of veins: superficial veins, located in the fatty tissue that lies just under the skin, and deep veins, located in the muscles. Deep-vein thrombosis is blood clotting in the deep veins of the legs. It usually occurs in the veins of the calf muscles. Although clotting can also occur in the superficial veins, DVT is more dangerous because all or part of the clot can break loose, travel along the bloodstream, and lodge in a narrow artery in the lung or another major organ, obstructing blood flow. A thrombus that moves is called an *embolus*.

A number of recognized factors can contribute to deep-vein thrombosis. Smoking, prolonged immobility, and (rarely) the contraceptive pill are a few of them. If a woman has Hughes syndrome, the chances of her developing a DVT during pregnancy increase, since the blood naturally becomes "stickier" during pregnancy. Once a patient has suffered one DVT, chances are he or she will have further episodes.

The number of people who became ill or even died after traveling by plane pushed DVT into the spotlight. The condition was dubbed *economy-class syndrome* by the media because it was widely thought that cramped conditions in the cabins of commercial aircraft contributed to or caused blood clots in individuals who flew on long trips. Indeed, when even a healthy person lies in bed or sits for an extended period of time, such as during recovery from surgery or for a lengthy trip by plane or car, the blood flow in the veins slows significantly. This happens because the calf muscles aren't contracting and squeezing the blood toward the heart. Slowing of the blood flow in the veins can contribute to DVT.

It took the tragic deaths of a number of otherwise healthy young passengers to create enough pressure on governments and airlines to look into airplane-cabin safety. Studies are underway into whether economy-class syndrome is a reality or simply a figment of an overexcited press. The airlines themselves are funding some of that research; it makes good business sense to be seen as doing something other than issuing vague warnings and support stockings. Perhaps it is surprising, then, that major airlines have as yet ignored compelling evidence that a good percentage of DVTs are likely the result of a person's having APS, a condition that is *exacerbated* by the cramped conditions in an aircraft cabin, but not *caused* by them. In Britain, the government has said that a review of cabin safety will include a look at DVT and APS.

Graham Hughes believes that if individuals who suffered DVTs after being on a commercial flight were tested for sticky blood, a significant percentage of them would turn up positive, possibly as many as one in four. He has seen a considerable number of patients who have had clots during or after flights and who tested positive for Hughes syndrome. To date, research into links between DVT and APS is limited, though in time, as more cases of this kind come to light, it may be possible to establish a firm connection. For airline passengers, this would be great news. It would give them a chance to prevent a DVT or to get treated quickly if they suffered one during or after a flight.

Dr. Hughes suggests that airline passengers should be given a simple questionnaire along with their ticket to assess their degree of risk for DVT. It would ask the following seven questions:

◆ Have you ever suffered a blood clot?

◆ Do you have recurrent migraine or severe headaches?

◆ Do you suffer from numbness in your fingers and toes?

- Do you have a family history of autoimmune disease?

- Have you had two or more miscarriages?

- Do you suffer memory loss or speech difficulties?

- Have you had treatment for poor circulation?

If a person answered yes to any of these questions, then an increased likelihood would exist that he or she had antiphospholipid syndrome, and the airline-issued questionnaire could recommend that he or she be screened for the illness. Identifying those who are at risk of having a DVT could prevent clots and save lives.

It is strongly advised that APS patients who travel by air get up and walk around the aircraft cabin every hour or two for a few minutes. If they're traveling by car, they should stop every hour or two and walk around outside the car for a few minutes.

Patients' Stories

Let's read about some individuals who suffered APS-related blood clots and were successfully treated for them.

* Jenny Dautlich

When Jenny Dautlich, a medical doctor, boarded a flight to New York three years ago, she had been diagnosed with a mild case of the autoimmune disorder lupus. She had also suffered a DVT in her leg thirteen years before, when she was twenty-eight, and had been treated with anticoagulants ever since. About the DVT, she recalls, "I was perfectly healthy, and then I got this terrible pain in my left leg. It was a large clot, and they decided to remove it. After that I was put on warfarin to thin my blood." Since she was taking the medication, it wasn't unreasonable for her to feel safe as she readied for her journey.

The years following the occurrence of her DVT had been unremarkable health-wise. In fact, Jenny had become frustrated with having to stay on medication when she felt well. She went to the hospital for tests in hopes that she could stop taking the warfarin. The results, however, were disappointing. "I didn't want to be on warfarin anymore, but the blood tests showed I needed it. The doctors thought I had lupus, but I was a borderline case. There was no mention of Hughes syndrome; I believe at the time no one at that hospital had heard of it."

When Jenny boarded the plane for the long flight to New York, she was on warfarin, but her INR was very low that day: 1.3 when it was normally 3 or 4. Jenny says the flight departure was moved forward: "They changed the time of my flight. I would have taken more warfarin if I'd had the time." It is unclear whether doing so would have made any difference in the near-fatal events that were to follow.

During the flight Jenny was fine—a little tired, but she put that down to the usual fatigue that accompanies travel. "I had been told to drink lots of water and take as much exercise as I could," she recalls. "I did both these things. I felt tired but nothing else."

The next day at her aunt's house in New York she began to feel very unwell. She felt as though her head were about to explode; the pain was devastating. She was dizzy and began vomiting. "I was having a bad headache; it was very strong. As a doctor I knew I was in trouble, but I was so confused and in such pain that it was difficult for me to fully understand what was happening. My brother-in-law is also a doctor, so the family called him. He told them to take me to the hospital as quickly as possible." Jenny's sister called a cab—luckily there was a large hospital nearby.

Jenny continues, "I remember being frustrated because in the emergency room the nurse was more concerned with writing down the details of my condition than with checking my blood pressure. When she did get around to doing my BP, it was dangerously low. It was then that the alarm bells started ringing in my head. I asked to see a doctor right away. Since I was one myself, I felt I could move things along, but the nurse didn't listen.

"I knew in my heart that I was very sick. I am a Christian so I began praying; then I took off my rings and my watch and gave them to my sister. I thought I was going to die. As they took me to another room, I told my sister not to cry and promised that I would be back, I just wasn't sure when. In truth, I didn't know if I could keep that promise. After that I fell into a coma."

Jenny had suffered a massive heart attack as well as a DVT. Once at the hospital, while she was being treated for the heart attack, she suffered a series of strokes. When she came around, her right side was paralyzed. She could not see or speak, and her right arm and leg were frozen.

Blood tests were done. That's when they told her she might have antiphospholipid syndrome. She says, "I had never heard of it, and there wasn't much information available, so I was in the dark. I didn't know what the diagnosis meant." In Jenny's case it very nearly meant death. But she pulled through and gradually recovered some of her health.

When Jenny was well enough to travel, she returned home. She continues taking anticoagulant medication to prevent a recurrence of a DVT. She has worked hard to get back some of what she lost. She says, "My right arm is still paralyzed, but I am learning to write again. I have seen a speech therapist. These days I can read again, but I still only have partial vision in my left eye." She has regained much of her speech. She still has flares, which are controlled by the anticoagulants. Determined to get on with her life, she is currently studying public health.

✳ Hilary Swarbrick

It was when Hilary Swarbrick was pregnant with her son in 1986 that she suffered her first clot in her leg. Treatment dealt with the clot, but her pregnancy was dogged by severe migraine attacks. Hilary had a history of these headaches, as well as circulation problems, varicose veins, and a discoloration of her feet.

"In 1989," she recalls, "I developed a DVT in my right leg and spent a week in the hospital on an intravenous heparin drip. When I was discharged, I was prescribed warfarin for three months and was told that the probable cause of the clot was the contraceptive pill I had been taking."

For the next five years, Hilary endured more symptoms without knowing what was wrong. She had bouts of phlebitis, a painful condition in which the veins repeatedly become inflamed due to clots. The migraines persisted, and she also suffered pain in her legs and chronic fatigue. Hilary became pregnant with her second child and at nine weeks developed another clot in her right leg. She was given heparin injections and was tested for lupus and Hughes syndrome. The results showed that her body was producing antiphospholipid antibodies (APLA).

At her thirty-week prenatal appointment, the doctor couldn't find the baby's heartbeat. A scan confirmed Hilary's worst fears: Her baby had died. She gave birth to Liam two days later. She was devastated. And things got worse. As she and her husband waited for their baby's body to be returned after a postmortem, she developed another DVT. After Liam's funeral she was admitted to the hospital. She later learned that the baby had died because clots had formed in the placenta, starving him of food and oxygen.

One day Hilary read an article about the work at St. Thomas' Hospital and made an appointment with Dr. Hughes. "After being diagnosed with Hughes syndrome, I felt so isolated and was in desperate need of information about my condition," she says. "I wanted to talk to someone who understood what I was going through, but there were few resources out there for people with the illness. To save others from going through the despair I felt, I decided to start an organization to offer support for people with APS. In January 1996, with the help of Ronnie Bray, I started the Hughes Syndrome Foundation."

Hilary also attended St. Thomas' Hospital's pregnancy clinic for those with APS. She continues, "In January 1997, I became pregnant again, and this time I was closely monitored by my doctor, the local hospital, and St. Thomas'. I attended a clinic regularly for blood tests, checkups, and Doppler blood-flow scans [see Chapter 3]. Although success wasn't guaranteed, I always came away from Dr. Hughes' clinic with a sense of optimism." In September, she gave birth by cesarean section to a healthy baby girl.

Hilary still has bouts of chronic tiredness, joint pain, and circulatory problems, but since starting the warfarin she no longer suffers migraine attacks or DVTs.

* Helene Heilpern

Travel is a big part of Helene Heilpern's life. She and her husband have homes in London and in the south of France, so they are always on the move. Helene also regularly travels to visit a close friend in Sri Lanka. The numerous long-haul flights had no effect on her health—until 2001.

"I had been on umpteen flights to Sri Lanka," Helen says. "My friend had lived there for three years, and I would see her often. Her husband is in the diplomatic service, so I would go to keep her company when he traveled.

"I never had a problem with the journey until my trip in 2001. There were some vacant seats next to mine, so I managed to lie down and sleep for most of the flight. I felt absolutely fine. My friend picked me up at the airport, and the next day we traveled to the seaside with her children. It was about five days after the flight that my left leg began to swell. I thought I had been bitten by something, and I wasn't too worried about it. I didn't see a doctor right away, but then the swelling increased. Two days later I saw a doctor who diagnosed cellulitis (a bacterial infection of the skin and the tissues just beneath the skin). He gave me some antibiotics and a stocking to wear, but the stocking was far too tight, because by now the swelling was so bad my leg was three times its normal size.

"The following week I was due to fly home. The doctor said that would be fine, but by the time I was scheduled to leave, I was having difficulty walking because my leg was so bad. I needed a wheelchair at the airport. When I got back to Britain, I was due to fly to Nice the next day to join my husband. I felt so unwell that my mother came to help me pack. When I arrived in Nice, I had to walk to the customs hall because they didn't have a wheelchair. It was agony. They even called my husband in to help me clear customs. He was angry with me for making the journey.

"The next day I saw a physician. Within minutes he had called an ambulance and I was on my way to the hospital. I was admitted to the intensive care unit. They did an ultrasound and found six clots in my leg."

Helene had no idea what danger she had been in. She still thought she was suffering from a bacterial infection, not deep-vein thrombosis. The French doctors treated her with strong anticoagulants to deal with the clots. That seemed to work well, and after a few days they gave her the all clear to go home.

Then, on the day she was due to leave the hospital, Helene experienced a terrible pain in her lower abdomen. "They did some tests and found cysts on my ovaries that were bleeding because of the anticoagulants," she says. "They had to operate to stop the bleeding. Fortunately the operation was a success and I was allowed to go home." These days Helene is on warfarin all the time, and when she flies, she uses support stockings.

Before this episode, Helene knew she had lupus. She had been diagnosed with it when she was just twenty years old, twenty-seven years before developing DVTs. At the time, she had just gotten married and was studying at the university to become a dietician. She developed several odd symptoms. "I was a complete mess," she recalls. "I couldn't control my body. My legs and arms would move around, and so would my tongue. I wouldn't speak to anyone because when I did try to talk, all that would come out was gibberish. I didn't speak to anyone about my symptoms for a month because I was so frightened by having no control. They put me on a massive dose of steroids. Then a doctor at my local hospital said he knew of a 'man who seemed to deal with this kind of disease.' So I went to see Dr. Hughes, and it is a tribute to him that I was well for twenty-seven years before I had the clots."

Helene was diagnosed with Hughes syndrome in 2001, and she is being treated with anticoagulants. It now seems likely that she suffered a stroke when she was twenty, although there is no way of knowing for sure. It is also likely that she developed Hughes syndrome over the years, in addition to the lupus. There are a growing number of cases like Helene's, wherein a patient who originally tested negative for APS but positive for lupus has in subsequent years tested positive for the antiphospholipid antibodies. It does not work the other way around, however. A person who has Hughes syndrome is very unlikely to later develop lupus.

* * *

As you can see from these case studies, blood clots are serious and require prompt treatment. Yet once identified, their recurrence can be prevented fairly easily with an appropriate course of blood thinners. The presence of a blood clot is one of the telltale signs of Hughes syndrome. In fact, a positive blood test for the antiphospholipid antibodies plus a clotting incident are considered definitive for diagnosing the disease (although some people test positive for the antibodies even though they have never suffered a blood clot).

Review the bulleted list of questions found earlier in this chapter (the ones that Dr. Hughes recommends should accompany airline tickets). If you answer yes to any of them, see your doctor and ask to undergo the blood tests for antiphospholipid antibodies. If your doctor exhibits doubt or a lack of awareness about APS, show him or her this book—or find a new doctor.

Chapter 3

Baby Blues

Any woman who has suffered a miscarriage knows what a lonely and devastating experience it can be. It is often made worse by the fact that those around her, including her doctor, will tell her not to worry and to try again as soon as her health allows. From a woman's point of view, miscarriage can seem like one of the harshest and most unsympathetic medical events.

Current medical wisdom says that the loss of one pregnancy is common and in general nothing to worry about, especially if it happens early in the pregnancy. This viewpoint also maintains that losing a second fetus is less common but also shouldn't cause undue concern. It is only when a woman suffers three miscarriages that the alarm bells start to ring and the medical machine kicks into action. The patient is told she suffers from "recurrent" or "habitual" miscarriage, and then the tests and investigations begin.

This system takes little account of how distressing even one miscarriage can be for a woman or couple wanting to start a family. The trauma of losing three or more babies is hard to imagine if it hasn't happened to you. It is a painful situation often compounded by the medical professionals' seeming disregard for the first two miscarriages. A considerable number of women who have experienced habitual miscarriage and to whom I spoke while researching this book felt that more could have been done sooner. They were convinced before the third miscarriage that there was an underlying problem that was going unaddressed. They struggled to be heard by their doctors and felt they were only taken seriously after they had suffered three miscarriages. In some cases that meant years of uncertainty or lack of knowledge about what was wrong.

Miscarriage and APS

What has this got to do with antiphospholipid syndrome? Miscarriage is one of the main clues that a woman might have the disorder. APS is responsible for as many as one in four cases of recurrent miscarriage. Graham Hughes is of the view that women should be tested for antiphospholipid antibodies after just one miscarriage, or even that the APS blood test should be part of routine prenatal screening. The test could be an early indicator that a woman needs special treatment in order to have a successful pregnancy, hopefully saving her the trauma of repeated miscarriage.

Anthony Kenny, M.D., obstetrician to the British royal family, believes that work in this field is groundbreaking. "The discovery that Hughes syndrome affects so many pregnant women is the most significant development in obstetrics in ten years," he says. "The implications for patients are tremendous. It means we can help prevent repeated miscarriage. It has given us an insight which we didn't have. This work has an enormous impact on the lives of those struggling to start a family."

Many women may have the antiphospholipid antibodies prior to pregnancy without knowing anything is wrong. It is only when they become pregnant that the condition makes its presence felt. When a woman is carrying a baby, her blood naturally becomes slightly more viscous or thick. Someone who also has Hughes syndrome is therefore much more likely to encounter problems carrying the baby to full term. One simple explanation for what happens is that the capillaries to the fetus from the placenta, which are fine and delicate, become blocked with clots, preventing the blood from getting to the fetus. Gradually the placenta withers, and the fetus fails to thrive and is aborted.

Treatment

If Hughes syndrome has been diagnosed in a pregnant woman, there is plenty that can be done to help. The drugs available are very effective and can be as mild as baby aspirin. Sometimes the blood thinner heparin is prescribed. It is given by self-administered injection, in the same way that a diabetic injects herself with insulin. Warfarin (brand name Coumadin), the most common prescription anticoagulant, is not prescribed during pregnancy or to women trying to get pregnant because it can cause birth defects.

In later pregnancy, women who are considered to be at risk are watched closely. The use of a *Doppler monitor* allows doctors to constantly observe the blood supply to the fetus. A Doppler test uses ultrasound (high-frequency sound waves that echo off the body) to examine blood flow. If the pulse begins to weaken or if signs indicate a reversal of blood flow, then an emergency cesarean section can be performed.

The success rate of treating women with APS who suffer recurrent miscarriage is greatly encouraging. At St. Thomas' Hospital, since the discovery of and improvements in treatment for the disorder, it has risen from under 20 percent to over 75 percent. Prior to these advances, a few of the patients at St. Thomas' pregnancy clinic had endured thirteen or more miscarriages; one woman had had more than twenty! The great news is that many of them have since enjoyed a happy ending—or perhaps I should say beginning.

Patients' Stories

✳ *Sharon Montgomery*

Sharon Montgomery was diagnosed with lupus when she was twenty years old. This was only after her doctor had dismissed her on a number of occasions, saying the symptoms were in her head. She endured joint pains, shortness of breath, and severe coughing. Eventually she saw a rheumatologist who immediately admitted her to the hospital; her heart had become enlarged and her kidneys were failing. With the right medication she pulled through but was in a wheelchair for months. She recovered well and got married the following year, to Adrian. She became pregnant, but sadly she miscarried early in the pregnancy.

"Four years later I became pregnant again," Sharon says. "I was delighted but anxious. My fears were confirmed when I miscarried at eight weeks. I was referred to a pregnancy clinic, where more tests were carried out."

She became pregnant and this time gave birth to a baby girl. But things were not right. Maxine was very premature and weighed only one pound. She was a fighter, but the odds were stacked against her and she died after three months.

The fact that she had given birth to a live baby gave Sharon and her husband hope that despite the difficulties they could realize their dream of starting a family. Sharon had two more miscarriages and then gave birth to a baby boy, whom they named Matthew. He was born at twenty-six weeks and weighed only one and a half pounds. Tragedy struck again and baby Matthew died after four days. To make matters even worse, Sharon became acutely ill after the birth and had to be rushed to the intensive care unit. She only saw Matthew once.

Sharon says, "I remember lying there and thinking how awful it was that it had happened again. I was devastated. I felt so ill and I couldn't help wondering why this kept happening to me. But it was worse for Adrian. He had to rush between Matthew and me because we were in two different hospital wards. He tried his best to keep tabs on both of us to make sure we were stable. He was so worried about us; it was such a terrible time for him. Words cannot describe the pain we felt when Matthew died. Adrian felt he never wanted to go through it all again. I could understand his feelings."

Eighteen months later the couple changed their minds. They decided to have one last try at starting the family they longed for. Because they had come so close, they felt there was a good chance of success. Under the guidance of a specialist who diagnosed

Sharon with Hughes syndrome and got her started on anticoagulant treatment, she was given daily injections of heparin and a weekly ultrasound. She was admitted to the hospital early and was cared for by a special midwifery team. At thirty-two weeks Sharon started to have problems with blood flow and blood pressure. Her baby was delivered by cesarean section.

Ben weighed in at three pounds. He was nicknamed Bam Bam in the pediatric-care unit because his initials were B.A.M.—but they just as easily could have been referring to his will to live. Ben might have been small, but he was strong. Sharon and Adrian's last gamble on having a child had paid off. "We went through so much in those years of trying for a child, and we came close to abandoning the whole thing," Sharon says. "I am so glad we didn't. Ben brings us such joy. He is now seven years old and full of life. He loves his school and enjoys music and dance. I can't imagine life without him." For Sharon and her husband, the pain of thirteen years of loss has melted away.

* Angela Steward

Angela Steward, once a product manager for a food manufacturer, was devastated when she was told her chances of having a baby were virtually nil. Angela, who's thirty-one, had suffered seven miscarriages. She was diagnosed after her third miscarriage with Hughes syndrome, but the treatment she received didn't help. Through sheer determination she finally found her way to the right medical team and got the medication that helped turn her dream of becoming a mom into a reality.

"When my little girl arrived, I couldn't stop crying," Angela says. "They were tears of utter joy. She was the miracle that I had longed for. I called her Jade because I read in a book that it meant 'a mother's most precious gift,' and she was certainly that to me.

"I had been trying for nine years to have a child, and I had lost seven babies. I decided I would have one last try. I couldn't keep putting my husband, David, and myself through the trauma of it all.

"We married young, when we were both twenty. About three years later we decided the time was right to have children. It's a cruel irony when you spend so many years of your life worrying that you might become pregnant by mistake. It never occurs to you that you might not be able to have children when you decide you want them.

"I remember being so thrilled when I was first pregnant. It was my mom and dad's twenty-fifth-anniversary party. My dad announced my pregnancy to everyone there, and he was beaming. We were too. Shortly after that I lost the baby. One of the hardest things was having to tell all these people that suddenly I wasn't pregnant anymore.

"I had gone for an ultrasound, which revealed that the baby had died at about ten and a half weeks but that the womb had kept on growing. It was awful. I waited a good year before trying again. But the same thing happened. That was disappointing, and it was even worse because they told me that until a woman has had three miscarriages, they wouldn't do any investigative work. I decided that I would get pregnant quite quickly the next time, because if there was a problem, I wanted them to find out what it was. I thought a lot about what was wrong with me, but the medical professionals said it was just the law of averages, the sort of thing that happened all the time. What can you do when they say that? You have to trust that they know better than you do.

"I suffered the third miscarriage, and the doctors started to do some tests. I had other hints that something was wrong. I was having symptoms like terrible, blinding headaches. My arms and legs were stiff and painful as well. I was only twenty-six, but I felt like an old woman. I would say this to my doctor and I was sure that he thought I was a hypochondriac.

"Finally a doctor brought to light that I might have a condition called Hughes syndrome. A blood test confirmed that I did, and I was put on injections of heparin and a daily dose of aspirin. I was desperate to know more, but there wasn't much information available.

"I was sent to a number of specialists, most notably a rheumatologist, but also a hematologist and a neurologist. Then I got pregnant again and my case was referred back to my obstetrician. It was so confusing and I felt so out of control, like I was being pushed around and nobody was really helping me. I lost the baby after ten weeks of pregnancy. I went on to get pregnant yet again, and to have yet another miscarriage, my fifth. I was devastated, and the pressure on us as a couple was dreadful. The whole thing was destroying our marriage. I felt as though I was a failure as a woman, that David should find a partner who could give him children. It was such a hard time for both of us.

"Then in December 1997, I read a newspaper article about a woman who had the same condition as I had. The treatment she'd received had helped her have a baby. The article mentioned the team at St. Thomas' Hospital in London. I knew that I had to see them, as they were specialists in this field. I didn't want to be fobbed off again. Getting a referral proved difficult, but at last it did come through.

"I got pregnant again. At seven weeks I was away from home giving a presentation for work, and I remember thinking, 'Should I be doing this?' The presentation went well, but the next day I began having a miscarriage. When I went to the hospital, they performed an ultrasound and said they had found a second heartbeat, which meant I was pregnant with twins. I thought, 'I can't cope with this roller coaster.' At the same time, I was elated by the news and hopeful that with the second twin things would be fine. But then, sadly, three weeks later, when we were on vacation, I had to be rushed to the hospital, where I lost the other twin. I think that was the worst miscarriage. I was very distressed.

"I seriously considered having a hysterectomy so I wouldn't have to keep going through all this, because it was taking over our lives. The team at St. Thomas' had made me realize that my chances for a successful pregnancy were slimmer than I had thought. They made me face reality that it was highly likely that I would be unable to carry a baby to term. This sounds odd, but I welcomed the news, that level of honesty. In the past I had been told I was just unlucky. They were the first people who understood what I was going through, and they talked straight to me, so I knew what to expect.

"At St. Thomas' I underwent more tests. I felt that I couldn't cope with an eighth miscarriage, but the doctors there said I should give it one last try. They put me on a different type of heparin and aspirin.

"When I got pregnant, I was monitored very closely both by St. Thomas' and by my local health-care team. It was a very diffi-cult pregnancy. I lost a lot of blood, and I was sure I would lose the baby. I can remember that at sixteen weeks, after another scare, I decided I couldn't do this any longer. I almost hoped they wouldn't find a heartbeat so it would be all over. I was numb when they did an ultrasound and said everything was fine.

"Jade was delivered by cesarean. The joy I felt was indescrib-able. People were worried about me because I was so high with it all. I was up and about really quickly. We were home after two days and I was so excited I couldn't sleep.

"I think if I hadn't pushed to see the right people I wouldn't have my beautiful baby or the happy and stable relationship with David that I have today. I would have given up on starting a family and thrown myself into my work.

"I would say to other women that they should look for the symptoms and refuse to be one of the herd. Every woman is so individual, and she has to make sure she is doing the best for her-self and her baby. Listen to the doctors, but if you have any doubts don't hesitate to get a second opinion. What happened to us is proof that it is worth fighting to get the right treatment."

✳ *Anna Divers*

Anna Divers, a systems development manager, was luckier than most because she was diagnosed with APS after only two miscar-riages. But she says she still found it tough to cope with the loss.

As she tells it, "I first became pregnant in August 1997. My husband and I were so overjoyed that we told everyone right away. At eight weeks I experienced a bit of spotting, so I went for an early ultrasound just to make sure everything was all right. Sure enough they found a heartbeat. But one week later the bleeding got heavier, and a second ultrasound showed no heartbeat, just an empty sac. I underwent a D and C to ensure that everything was removed and to prevent infection. That was it—no advice, no counseling. We were told this was very common. That didn't help us at all. We were devastated; it had never crossed our minds that such a thing might happen to us. I threw myself into work as a way of coping. We didn't have the courage to try again for three years.

"In July 2000, I became pregnant again. This time we told no one; we were scared it might all go wrong again. And it did. I miscarried at nine weeks with exactly the same symptoms: one week of spotting, an ultrasound showing that all was well, then the next week nothing.

"I was convinced this wasn't just 'one of those things.' I thought that something might be wrong with the environment the baby was trying to grow in, even though I had lived like a nun this time around. I felt stronger than I had after the first miscarriage. I was determined to find out why this had happened, even though I knew that doctors don't normally investigate the cause of miscarriages until you've suffered the agony of three. By chance I saw a different doctor, and she suggested I go for a blood test. I was found to have the antiphospholipid antibody, which I was told caused the blood to become 'sticky' and in pregnancy made the blood flow through the placenta poorly, creating problems for the growing fetus."

Anna was referred to a gynecologist who specialized in APS-related pregnancy problems. She became pregnant in April 2001 and was put on daily injections of heparin and low-dose aspirin, both prescribed to thin the blood.

She says, "I was fortunate enough to attend the fetal medicine unit at the hospital, and that gave me tremendous reassurance.

The doctors prescribed ultrasounds early, at six weeks. When they did the second one, at seven weeks, we heard one of the team say, 'How many did we see last week?' That confused us completely. Then we realized there were two heartbeats—we were having twins.

"I'm not religious, but it seemed almost as if having twins was somehow making up for the two I had lost before. After that, I said a prayer every day of my pregnancy.

"On December 12, Harry and Jack arrived. I was proud that they were delivered normally and that I had carried them to thirty-nine weeks. They were excellent weights: six pounds thirteen ounces, and five pounds ten ounces. I am certain this was because the blood flow through the placenta was so good due to the treatment I was on.

"I still can't believe the twins are here. I owe so much to the doctor who sent me for the simple blood test that made the successful pregnancy possible and gave us Harry and Jack."

* Maria Pepe

When Maria first became pregnant, she was thirty-six years old and in good health. She was fit, active, and under no particular stress. As she remembers the events, "Everything went well up to week twenty-nine of the pregnancy. It was then that I became aware that I hadn't felt the baby move for a day or so. I wasn't particularly worried as he wasn't much of a kicker anyway, but we went to the hospital for reassurance. Unfortunately we got a shock: The baby had died."

The postmortem showed that the placenta had sheared away from the womb, but it wasn't clear why that had happened. Several tests revealed nothing, until the results came back from one of Maria's blood tests. It showed she carried the antiphospholipid antibodies. The doctors thought this condition could have caused a blockage in the placenta, leading to the death of her baby.

Maria continues, "The next year, I became pregnant again and was referred to a specialist in treating Hughes syndrome pregnancies. He recommended aspirin and an injection of heparin daily to thin my blood. I also underwent regular ultrasounds to monitor the blood flow to and from the placenta. The pregnancy went well, and three weeks ahead of time our son was born by cesarean. He arrived weighing six pounds four ounces and in radiant health. It was wonderful."

Notice that one of the common threads running through these women's stories is how they had to persist to find the right doctor and to get the right diagnosis and treatment for their recurrent miscarriages. As Angela says, listening to the doctors is important, but it's equally important to trust your hunches and obtain a second opinion if you have doubts about what you're being told by any medical professional.

Of all the topics covered in this book, this is the one that brings the most hope and good news. For the relatively small cost and effort of monitoring for Hughes syndrome in the early stages of pregnancy, many women and families could be saved the agony of repeated miscarriages. Regarding whether such preventive procedures should be covered by insurance, the insurance companies should consider how much they would save if the number of miscarriages suffered later in pregnancy, with their costly medical expenses, was reduced by as much as 75 percent.

Chapter 4

Stroke

Stroke is one of the biggest killers in developed countries. In the United States someone suffers a stroke every fifty-three seconds. It is also one of the most costly conditions, as individuals who survive a stroke often need a good deal of medical care. It is the largest single cause of severe disability. The annual cost of treating stroke patients is considerable, estimated at $3.6 billion in the United Kingdom and a massive $36 billion in the United States.

When people think of a stroke victim, they imagine an older person, probably someone who has had a lifetime of physical neglect, who has indulged in too many cigarettes and a bad diet, gotten no exercise, and has been subjected to too much stress. But the reality is that anyone, young or old, can suffer a stroke. We've all heard stories of the man in his mid-thirties who doesn't smoke, watches his weight, and exercises regularly, but who collapses on the squash court with a stroke.

APS Implicated in Stroke

In simple terms, a stroke is the death of brain tissue resulting from an interruption in the blood flow and insufficient oxygen to the brain. Although there are some well-known causes of stroke, such as high blood pressure, in most cases doctors do not know what triggers one. Strokes are classified as either *ischemic* or *hemorrhagic*.

An ischemic stroke occurs when the blood supply to the brain is cut off because either atherosclerosis (the accumulation of fatty material inside the walls of the arteries) or a blood clot has blocked a blood vessel. A hemorrhagic stroke occurs when a blood vessel bursts, inhibiting normal blood flow and allowing blood to leak into a part of the brain and destroy it. In APS-related stroke, the blood thickens and clots, cutting off supply to parts of the brain, starving the area of oxygen, and leading to an ischemic stroke.

A study of stroke patients in Spain showed that 7 percent had Hughes syndrome. Further work by a team in Rome looked at so-called young strokes, those occurring in people under the age of forty-five. The results showed that 16 percent of such patients had the antiphospholipid antibody. The conclusion drawn from these data is that as many as one in five strokes involving people age forty and under is due to Hughes syndrome.

Graham Hughes and his team regard this discovery as highly significant. The findings bring fresh hope to victims and potential victims of stroke. Establishing a new identifiable cause of strokes means that some cases can be treated more effectively using anticoagulants to thin the blood. It also means that in people who are thought to be at risk of having Hughes syndrome, such as those who have suffered thrombosis or severe headaches, it may be possible to prevent a stroke from happening by performing blood tests and treating positive results. Even when there is no previous medical history of APS symptoms, if a young person has a stroke, Dr. Hughes believes he or she should be tested for APS as a matter of course. If the stroke victim does carry the antibody, then further strokes could potentially be prevented and the damage done by the stroke could be limited.

Patients' Stories

* *James Dorrington-Ward*

James Dorrington-Ward is a perfect example of how stroke can suddenly happen out of nowhere, even in a young and apparently healthy person. When he was eighteen, James decided to take a year off and travel across South America with a group of friends. For him it was to be the trip of a lifetime to be taken before putting his head down and working hard at college. The group had already been to Chile and Bolivia; their next plan was to tackle the Inca Trail, which would take them to a summit fourteen thousand feet above sea level.

They had been at ten thousand feet for a month before starting on the trail, so they all, including James, were well acclimatized. However, as they made their way higher and higher, James became more and more fatigued. He blamed himself for not eating and drinking properly; he put his tiredness down to being terribly unfit. But it wasn't the lack of training that was leaving him gasping for air.

"On the second day we were going up a steep climb," he says. "I was hot, but there was a cold wind, so I couldn't take off any clothes despite the fact that I was sweating badly. I was struggling for breath and felt incredibly tired. I just thought I was out of shape. It got to the point where the others were pushing me up; it was embarrassing. We got to a plateau at lunchtime. I couldn't eat or drink even though I was thirsty. I just wanted to sleep.

"There were only four hundred feet to go to reach the top, but it was very, very steep. The others went on ahead, as they could see I was in bad shape. The guide stayed with me. I started walking the last bit, fifty steps at a time. I managed three sets and then I fell to the ground. I was completely disoriented and I remember wondering why I couldn't feel my left side. It was as though that part of my body had just shut down, although I felt no pain in my side or in my head. Once again I just thought it was due to tiredness. I had been suffering from altitude sickness for some time before the climb. I was helped up and I recovered enough to sit on a rock. I still couldn't feel my left side. It wasn't frightening because I didn't understand then what was happening. Some of my strength came back, and I got angry with myself for letting the others down. I forced myself to get to the top.

"On the way down I had to use a stick, as I was limping. We went down to 13,500 feet, where the camp was located. I had about 50 percent mobility in my left leg. I went to bed and slept. But I woke in the night to find my body shaking violently. I was having the first of many epileptic fits. I couldn't move or speak. The seizure lasted about five minutes."

The next morning, the porters had to carry James down the next part of the trail to where there were donkeys that could take him to the bottom of the mountain. "I kept having more shakes, and I had a huge seizure," he recalls. "It was then that I began to feel afraid. I thought, 'Oh my God, I can't control this.' " But James noticed that he began to feel better as soon as he was no longer at high altitude.

Once off the trail he was taken to a small local hospital, admitted as an emergency patient, and put on an IV drip. Facilities were limited, so he was moved to a larger hospital in Lima where a CT scan was performed. The doctors suspected that James had suffered a stroke, but the scan showed nothing. The priority was to get him home. There, James again went to the hospital, where they did an MRI scan, which revealed lesions or white marks on his brain. "I was told that I had suffered a stroke and had a form of lupus," he says. "I was put on high-dose warfarin injections. But my family and I weren't happy with the diagnosis. We felt it wasn't accurate. I was lucky that my uncle, who is a doctor, knew a specialist and arranged for me to see him. At the time, I hadn't heard of APS. It certainly wasn't something the doctors at my local hospital knew about."

Blood tests showed that James did not have lupus. Instead, they revealed that he carried the antiphospholipid antibodies. He had Hughes syndrome. His stickier-than-normal blood and the extremely high altitude triggered the stroke and seizures. At great heights it becomes more difficult to get oxygen into the blood. (James didn't become ill when he was traveling in an aircraft at high altitudes because aircraft cabins are pressurized.) If James had not gone on that trek, he might never have learned that he had this condition.

James says about his diagnosis, "I was relieved, because I realized that Hughes syndrome wasn't as bad as lupus. I didn't have to have the warfarin injections. Instead I was prescribed simple aspirin. And it worked."

Five years later James is still taking aspirin and has had no recurrence of stroke or seizures. He is currently working to qualify as an accountant and says he is so well that he finds it hard to believe what happened to him on that hostile mountainside in Peru.

According to Graham Hughes, cases like James's, where there were no previous medical problems, are unusual, although he has seen children as young as four who have suffered a stroke and subsequently test positive for APS. In James' case the doctors assume that the tendency toward APS had been present for some time, and that the conditions at high altitude tipped the balance into an actual blood clot.

* Janine Billet

More common than James' situation are those of patients who have a long history of illness and who suffer what are known as "warning" strokes. In some cases they might not even realize they have suffered a series of strokes until a brain scan is carried out following other symptoms. Such was the case with Janine Billet. Janine had endured a lifetime of illness. When she was only ten, she began suffering from severe headaches followed by aching muscles and joints. Doctors dismissed these problems as growing pains, but they didn't go away when she stopped growing; they just got worse.

Now Janine is forty-five, and her medical history charts years of suffering and uncertainty. Although she has two healthy children who are in their twenties, she had five miscarriages before age twenty-six. She suffered numerous episodes of painful deep-vein thrombosis in her arms and legs. She continued to have head-aches, and she also endured severe internal bleeding that led to an early hysterectomy. To make matters worse, for most of her life she did not know what was wrong.

Despite all these setbacks Janine was a fighter, determined not to give in to her illness. She had always had an agile brain. She started her career as a bookmaker's settler, a job that required her to quickly add up figures. As the years went by, she began to notice that she was slowing down. "I found that I got befuddled with fig-ures," she says. "I decided to work for myself as a market trader. And then my grasp of words was affected. My daughter would laugh when I would tell her to 'get the umbrella from the drawer' when I meant knife.

"I have always enjoyed doing crosswords in the newspapers. I found the one in the local paper so easy that I would rocket through it, solving the clues as quickly as I could write the answers. *The New York Times* crossword took a bit more time, but it was rare that I hadn't finished it by lunchtime." As her condition worsened, however, she found that not only did she have difficulty getting the answers, she could hardly read and understand the clues. Janine knew something was terribly wrong but had no idea what it might be.

Despite not knowing what was behind her deteriorating mind, Janine would not be beaten. She decided to return to school to study psychology. In her first year, when she was thirty-three years old, she had a stroke. "It was the worst thing that had happened to me," she recalls. "It left me weak on one side, and it permanently damaged my peripheral vision. It robbed me of a lot of my vocabu-lary. I found it difficult to write the papers assigned for school, because although I knew the words I wanted to use, I couldn't get them out. My tutors would point out that I had written the exact opposite of what I meant. Luckily they were very supportive. I had only completed one term and everyone thought that would be it, that I would have to give up my studies. But the university was very helpful and encouraged me to take my exams. No one expected me to get through it, including myself. I was flabbergasted when I passed. That proved to me that I should carry on as normal. I was determined to finish the program.

"It was quite a moment for me when I got the degree with honors. I had succeeded. I am a positive person and I believe that is what helped me reach my goal."

Ill health had dogged Janine as she struggled through school. "It was exceptionally hard. I had difficulty breathing, and I had serious chest pains," she says. "After leaving the university I ended up in a wheelchair unable to do much for myself. My memory was appalling. I forgot how to do basic things like switch on a TV or a washing machine. I was being admitted to the hospital on a regular basis at this point. I had what the doctors believed was a pulmonary embolism. When I survived it, they said I must have an angel on my shoulder.

"By early 1997, I was becoming desperate to find out what was wrong with me. I was seeing a number of doctors in different areas of medicine—a neurologist, urologist, ophthalmologist, and cardiologist, to name but a few. Each one was treating the symptoms in isolation. It was suggested I had chronic fatigue syndrome or multiple sclerosis. Not one of the physicians looked at the whole picture. It was suggested I was a hysterical patient. Out of desperation, I agreed to see a psychiatrist. He assured me that my problems were definitely medical, although he was surprised that I wasn't suffering from reactive depression triggered by the lack of support I had received. He referred me to yet another specialist, this time one who treated antiphospholipid syndrome. It was the best thing anyone could have done.

"I arrived at the clinic in a wheelchair. I was a very sick woman. To my utter relief, the doctor did not invalidate my symptoms. He understood what was wrong, and for the first time in years I had some hope. After my first consultation I began to see light at the end of the tunnel. Tests were done which showed I had Hughes syndrome. I was treated with anticoagulants. Gradually I found it easier to breathe, and my memory began to return. After a few months the wheelchair was stored away and I used the elevator less and less."

For the first time as an adult, Janine enjoyed some quality of life and felt hopeful for her future. These days she is racing through the crosswords again. If she finds they become difficult, she knows it is a sign that her condition is flaring up and that she needs to increase her medication.

* Lynda Smock

Lynda Smock had a stroke in May 2001, an event that puzzled the doctors in her hometown in Arizona. Lynda was forty, didn't smoke or drink, had low blood pressure, and was only marginally overweight. She says, "I had the stroke at home, and all the doctors I saw just shrugged their shoulders and said they didn't know why it had happened to me. I was told to take one aspirin a day and I would be fine."

"A few weeks later," she continues, "I had a second, much bigger stroke. That got their attention! In the emergency room, I lay in my bed and prayed for God to send the right doctor to me. I refused to tell them the name of my neurologist because I thought he was an idiot. So the team at the hospital brought in a specialist who literally saved my life. He asked if he could test for a special disease that caused migraines and miscarriages in early life, and strokes and heart attacks later on. I have two healthy teenagers, but I did have three miscarriages when I was younger, and I had a history of migraines. Furthermore, I was hospitalized with a blood disorder when I was six."

Lynda agreed to undergo blood tests. They showed she had APS. She was given anticoagulants and appeared to recover. Five months later she was taken off the medication in preparation for a surgical procedure. As a result, she says, "I had a third stroke. They simply hadn't given me enough heparin to prevent it in the days preceding the operation." Lynda's doctors increased her dose of heparin, and the symptoms of the stroke mostly disappeared, leaving her with only minimal memory damage and some tiring on her right side.

Although relieved to finally be able to attach a name to her problems, and grateful for the recovery she's experienced, Lynda finds it hard to avoid worrying about the implications of this serious condition. "My children now live with the worry that Mom might have a stroke and not recover," she says. "They call me throughout the day to make sure I am okay. It is a shame they no longer have the innocence and confidence they should have, because their mom isn't 'Supermom' anymore. I get tired and cranky, whereas before I was the most patient soul around. My husband is concerned that I won't live to see my grandbabies. I probably won't have any for ten to twelve years, but I want to be there for my children and to help them celebrate a new generation of life."

Lynda is convinced that Hughes syndrome runs in her family. Once she got a diagnosis, she began to retrace her relatives' medical history, and she feels certain the condition has been responsible for deaths in three generations of her family. She says, "My grandfather William was bedridden for the last two years of his life with horrid headaches and partial paralysis on one side. His death certificate says he was killed by a brain tumor, but we wonder if it was antiphospholipid syndrome. This happened back in 1939, in Kentucky, so there is no way we could ever be sure. My mom died of an apparent heart attack at fifty-five. Yet we have no other history in the family of heart disease. Mom had been to the hospital twice with headaches, chest pains, and extreme fatigue. Tests on her heart showed that it was fine. Looking back, I think a blood clot was the culprit, because the coroner said the heart had been starved of oxygen.

"Then my brother Michael died of a stroke in his sleep when he was forty-four. No one could understand why. Perhaps it was caused by an APS-related clot." Lynda intends to watch for symptoms of Hughes syndrome that might indicate the existence of the condition in the next generation of her family. She and her husband plan to have tests done on their children to see if they carry the antibody.

About learning to live with her health problems, she says, "Without a strong faith in God and a family to laugh with and help me through the tough times, I think I would have gone mad and given up. These days I am constantly cautious about what I eat and do. In the face of this disease, my life has changed forever."

✳ ✳ ✳

Two points from the stories included in this chapter deserve to be highlighted. First, notice how Janine uses her ability to complete the daily crossword puzzle as a gauge to tip her off about whether her dose of anticoagulant needs to be adjusted. To reiterate something Dr. Hughes noted earlier in this book, APS patients, especially those who experience neurological symptoms, seem to "know" when their medication level is right. It's important that you learn to trust your body and your hunches about your condition—and then insist on being taken seriously by the medical professionals to whom you've entrusted your care.

Second, in Lynda's case, the doctors stopped her regimen of anticoagulants to prepare her for a surgical operation—a standard precautionary measure observed when anyone who takes blood thinners is planning to undergo surgery. The result for Lynda of going off her blood thinner even for a short time? She suffered another stroke. APS experts and advocates emphasize the importance for APS patients of taking very seriously any suggestion that they suspend their anticoagulant therapy. A pamphlet written by two APS patients addresses the issue as follows:[2]

> If you have had a blood clot (or any other medical condition caused by a clot—e.g., stroke, heart attack) and have tested positive for APS, do not ever, under any circumstances, let a doctor take you off of a blood thinner without seeing a doctor familiar with APS for a second opinion. It is necessary, at times, to change the type of blood thinner when required for surgical or dental procedures....

Some doctors will treat you with blood thinners for six months and then take you off the thinners "to see what happens." I can tell you what will happen—a very high probability that you will have another clot. The clot can easily result in a heart attack or stroke. However, if the disease is treated correctly, life should be near normal and your life expectancy is probably as good as anyone else's.

Once again, as these stories make clear, and especially in the face of the lack of awareness about Hughes syndrome among the general medical community, APS patients must act as their own best advocates.

Chapter 5

Headaches

After talking to many patients with antiphospholipid syndrome, one is struck by the fact that the single most common symptom they suffer from is recurrent, severe headaches. We all have headaches from time to time, but in people with sticky blood, these can be a warning sign that something else is wrong.

APS: A Pain in the Head?

Imagine the fine capillaries in the brain becoming clogged, or the blood flow to the brain being restricted because the blood is too thick. Both of these scenarios are conceivable in individuals with Hughes syndrome, and you can see why either of them might cause a pain in the head. Because a headache isn't usually something that makes a person rush to the doctor's office, most people who get a headache take a few painkillers and forget about it. However, in those with Hughes syndrome, headache could be the first indicator that the disease is present. Many APS patients say they began to have headaches when they were teenagers, and the pain became an untreated feature of their lives. It was only later that they developed other aspects of APS. There is also evidence that women may suffer APS-related headache during or after pregnancy, when their blood is already naturally thicker because of the pregnancy.

In a large number of cases that arrive at the clinic in St. Thomas' Hospital, the headaches are accompanied by other symptoms, such as flashing lights, nausea, and vomiting. Migraine sufferers will recognize these unpleasant features. At present there is no cure for true migraine, although an array of drugs is available to relieve the symptoms. If, however, it is Hughes syndrome that has triggered the migraine, then it is possible to treat and prevent it.

Graham Hughes predicts that antiphospholipid syndrome will become an important recognized cause of migraine, but because it is still a relatively new disease, at this time there has been little research into this link. The Rayne Institute at St. Thomas' Hospital has conducted a trial to determine if anticoagulation drugs help Hughes syndrome patients who suffer debilitating headaches. The results are impressive: People with intractable migraine say the pain disappears once the drugs are started.

Such findings could have broad implications for the treatment of headache, and of migraine in particular. It will be necessary, though, to push for more research to verify these early findings. For now, the best witnesses to this "miracle" cure are the patients themselves.

Patients' Stories

✳ *Jaine Foster*

Jaine Foster had never suffered badly from headaches until her second pregnancy. She did, however, have a history of illness. Diagnosed with rheumatoid arthritis when she was sixteen, she developed deformities of some joints and needed corrective surgery. The drugs she was prescribed to treat the arthritis proved ineffective, and it wasn't until she was twenty-one that tests showed she actually suffered from lupus. The lupus had gone untreated and therefore had caused damage that Jaine feels could have been avoided if she'd received an earlier diagnosis. But twenty-two years ago doctors didn't generally look for lupus, never mind Hughes syndrome.

Like many sufferers of lupus and APS, Jaine had problems getting pregnant, so she and her husband decided to try in vitro fertilization (IVF). It worked, and they had a baby daughter, Jasmine. Four years later the couple tried for their second child. It was while she was pregnant with Oliver that Jaine experienced the worst, most grueling pain she has ever known.

"At fifteen weeks I started to get a very bad headache," she says. "It was an intense pain, but worst of all nothing seemed to stop it. I went to the pharmacist and asked for everything and anything to stop my head from hurting. I tried relaxation tapes, reflexology, headache pills, migraine pills, stress-relief pills, but it was no good; the nightmare just went on. It felt as though I were wearing a skullcap that was far too tight. The pain was there when I went to sleep and when I woke up. I became desperate. I kept thinking that it would never go away, that I would always feel this bad.

"As I got nearer to my due date, I comforted myself with the thought that the pregnancy was the cause of the headache and that once I had given birth it would go away and let me get on with my life. I had Oliver, and sure enough it did leave. I was delighted."

Her joy was to be short-lived. Two weeks later the headache returned with a vengeance. The pain was so severe that it robbed Jaine of her ability to enjoy her new baby. With a young daughter and a new baby to care for, she was under enormous pressure. Her husband did what he could, but Jaine became depressed at the seemingly incurable pain in her head. "I cried a lot at that time," she recalls. "I had this baby who wouldn't sleep and a head that wouldn't stop hurting. It was pounding and pounding. I thought, 'I am supposed to enjoy this baby, who cost a fortune because of the IVF, and instead my world is crumbling.'

"I really thought my world was coming to an end; it felt as though everything was falling apart around me. I got to the point where I knew I couldn't cope. My husband would come home from work, and he would take over and let me go to bed. But even as I went to sleep, I knew the pain would be there when I awoke. It was dreadful.

"I thought I should be over the moon with happiness, but instead I couldn't cope anymore. I often called the team at the lupus clinic for support, and they were helpful, but it didn't take away the pain. I just wanted to curl up and die."

The headache was not like a migraine; Jaine says her eyes were not affected. Rather, the pain was all over her head, like a bonnet. Painkillers and other treatments made no difference. Richard decided that a weekend away by the seaside might help. Jaine was reluctant to go because she felt so unwell. Before the trip she went to see Dr. Hughes.

Jaine had been tested a number of times for the antiphospholipid antibody. One test was positive; the other two were negative. So she wasn't sure whether or not she had Hughes syndrome. Dr. Hughes decided to put her on a course of heparin injections. Because she had been through IVF twice, Jaine knew how to inject herself in the stomach.

The family went on their trip, and Jaine began the medication. "I remember looking at Richard as I injected myself and saying, 'Look, yet another needle,' because I had taken so many injections for the IVF." Jaine had no idea if the heparin would work, but she was desperate enough to try anything. She says at one point she literally banged her head hard against a wall just to see if doing so relieved the pain. Needless to say, it didn't.

After giving herself the shot, she says, "I woke the next day with this terrible feeling that something was missing. I panicked and went to check on the kids. They were fine, so I started pacing around the room trying to remember what it was that I had misplaced. Then it dawned on me: I no longer had the headache. It was completely gone. It was brilliant; the sense of relief I felt is hard to describe. It was sheer joy not to have that grinding pain in my head anymore. I felt that at last I could get on with my life."

Jaine says it took a few more days for the heparin to eliminate the headache completely. When the course of heparin was finished, the pain came back, so she had to continue with anticoagulant medication. In the two years since, Jaine has been mostly headache free. She was put on warfarin, which is taken orally, so she would no longer have to inject herself. With a home-test kit, she keeps a close watch on her INR (internationally normalized ratio; see Chapter 12). If it falls too low, she knows the headache will return. And if it does return, these days she also knows there is an end to the pain. Drugs exist that can help, which means she doesn't have to resort to hitting her head against a brick wall.

✳ Jason Abosch

After hearing about this book, Jason got in touch with me via the Internet. He said he wanted to share his story. When you have a chronic disease, it helps to know you are not alone; isolation and illness are tough to live with. Sometimes simply telling others what you have been through helps you cope with the daily ups and downs of a condition such as Hughes syndrome.

Twenty-four-year-old Jason was in excellent health. He worked out six times a week at his local gym in Baltimore, studying karate. Then in November 2000, his world collapsed.

One morning, he says, "I woke up with a terrible headache. Prior to that, I never got headaches. It gradually got worse during the day, and by noon I noticed that my vision was beginning to falter. My vision continued to deteriorate, the headache persisted, and then all of the sudden I had numbness. The numbness began in my arm, proceeded to my leg, and then made its way up to my cheeks, chin, and tongue. I also began losing the use of my right hand, was speaking slowly and in a confused manner, and suffered some short-term memory loss. I was definitely scared. Until then, I had been in excellent physical health. I knew something was not right. I called my physician and saw him later that day."

Unlike the vast majority of patients in this book, Jason was fortunate enough to get a diagnosis very quickly. Although his doctor was in the dark about Hughes syndrome, Jason saw a neurologist who was familiar with the condition and recognized the symptoms. "It took two weeks to diagnose," he says. "I underwent MRI and CT scans. They gave me a spinal tap and did a lot of blood tests. The blood work revealed the condition. It was some-what difficult for my physicians to diagnose—this was a rather unknown condition to them. Fortunately, I saw a neurologist who was well read, and he knew enough about the condition to test me for it. He, in all likelihood, saved my life. Except for the blood test, all the other tests were normal. My symptoms could have easily been dismissed as a freak occurrence."

Jason found it difficult to deal with the sudden change from being a fit young man to taking a cocktail of medication and being stalked by a fickle and unpredictable illness. He says, "Having this condition has changed my life. After diagnosis, I spent five days in the stroke unit at a hospital. For a twenty-four-year-old, that is emotionally tough. It is a condition I wrestle with rather routinely. My diet has changed dramatically, and I have to be cautious in my daily activities. I get headaches all the time, and stress has a greater effect on me.

"I have spent a total of fifteen days or so in the hospital in the last thirteen months. I take a handful of pills each day. And the condition also puts stress on my girlfriend and other family mem-bers. There are a lot of little things that I needed to change, and in the aggregate they have had a profound effect on everyday life.

"My blood is tested every two weeks. I take five medications: Coumadin (the brand name for the anticoagulant warfarin), vera-pamil (for headaches), baby aspirin, Imitrex (for headaches), and stool softener (due to the side effects cause by verapamil). I see a specialist at Johns Hopkins Hospital every six months, and I con-sult with a neurologist and physician when I need to. To deal with the emotional aspect of the changes in my life, I also visited with a psychiatrist for a few months after diagnosis."

For Jason the diagnosis of APS was devastating, and he is struggling to cope with being unwell. "Things are still much like a roller coaster," he says. "I have reminders of the condition each day—sometimes it's headaches, or not being able to eat something or do something, or even just taking medication. The thickness of my blood fluctuates a lot, so the levels of my medications often change. The biggest day-to-day problem is headaches and, occasionally, blurred vision. All of that being said, I consider myself fortunate. This condition is more of an inconvenience then anything else. There are other medical issues that are ten times worse."

Jason's attitude echoes what many people with Hughes syndrome say about the disease: true, the illness changes your life in ways that can bring stress and may seem unfair. Yet, once it's been diagnosed and treatment has begun, because the therapy is so simple and usually so effective, it's fairly easy to keep it all in perspective and even to feel grateful that things aren't worse.

Chapter 6

Do You Really Have Multiple Sclerosis?

One of the most alarming aspects of Hughes syndrome is how easily it can be mistaken for other conditions. As more cases come to light, it is clear that APS is often overlooked. This isn't a criticism of doctors who fail to spot it; it is simply a reflection of the current lack of awareness about the condition. If you are not looking for it, chances are you won't find it.

MS or APS?

Perhaps the most dramatic example of this phenomenon is in relation to multiple sclerosis. At this time, no one knows how often Hughes syndrome is mistaken for MS, because little research into the matter has been undertaken. But a closer look at the cases of mistaken identity is likely to reveal that the numbers are significant. In one recent clinic that specialized in autoimmune disease, in particular lupus, Graham Hughes saw three patients who had been told they had MS but whose blood tests showed they were actually suffering from APS. There were about forty patients at that clinic; a quick bit of mental math shows that just under 10 percent had mistakenly been told they had MS. Obviously, that figure could be irrelevant beyond the patients who found their way to this particular clinic. But a growing body of evidence supports the premise that the numbers of people misdiagnosed could be large; therefore, the pressure for greater knowledge is increasing.

How could it happen that a blood-clotting disease is sometimes mistaken for a disorder of the nervous system such as multiple sclerosis? Recall from Dr. Hughes' sidebar in Chapter 1 (pages 14–17) that the brain is especially vulnerable to the thickening or clotting of the blood caused by APS. When the brain is starved of oxygen, one of the predictable responses includes neurological symptoms that mimic those of MS. For more about how these symptoms might manifest themselves in APS, read the patients' stories below.

The difference for the patient between MS and APS could not be more profound. Both diseases are incurable and can result in debilitating symptoms. But a number of crucial distinctions exist between the two. MS is a progressive, degenerative illness that eats away at the nervous system. It is characterized by the destruction of the myelin sheath surrounding the nerves in the brain, spinal cord, and eyes. The myelin sheath is a sort of "insulation" that coats every nerve fiber. When myelin is damaged, nerves lose their ability to conduct impulses properly. Therefore, MS patients face the prospect of losing their mobility, becoming confined to a wheelchair, and suffering slurred speech, muscle weakness, double vision, and generalized numbness, all of which can get worse throughout their lives. The damage done is often permanent. Despite the disability, however, most people with MS have a normal life span. There is no fully acknowledged treatment for MS, although beta-interferon is believed to slow the progress of the disease. The best weapon a patient has is knowledge and courage.

On the other hand, although being told you have Hughes syndrome is not good news, in most cases the outlook is nowhere near as tough as it is for MS. Once a patient gets over the shock of the diagnosis and learns a little more about this relatively unknown condition, then the general picture is more promising. Most important to remember is that APS is extremely treatable. Unlike for MS, a number of highly effective, inexpensive prescription drugs are readily available for APS. And in some cases a prescription isn't required; the disorder can be controlled with baby aspirin. The damage caused is usually temporary, and with the right monitoring, the patient can expect to lead a relatively normal life.

How Often Is APS Misdiagnosed? A Look at One Study

Over the years doctors in this field have shared a growing concern about how common the misdiagnosis of MS for APS might be. The team at St. Thomas' decided to analyze a sample of patients stored in their records. Their research paper was published in 2000, and the result was enough to raise even the most cynical eyebrow.

The research group at the hospital's Rayne Institute, led by Dr. Maria Cuadrado, looked at the cases of twenty-seven women patients who had been originally diagnosed either as having MS or as most likely having MS. They had all attended the clinic over a period of two years. For most of the patients, a primary reason for the initial diagnosis was that their MRI (magnetic resonance imaging) brain scans showed lesions. In lay terms, lesions are ominous white "blobs" that appear on the scan. (The scan itself looks like an X ray of the brain, but an MRI isn't an X ray. Rather than using radiation, the MRI procedure derives its images by generating a very powerful magnetic field.) If a doctor refers to "white matter" in reference to an MRI scan, she or he is talking about white blobs that aren't supposed to be there. The blobs are one of the major abnormalities doctors look for when they suspect MS. But white spots on an MRI scan can also indicate the sort of blood clots that result from APS. For all the patients in this study, the devastating news that they had, or most likely had, MS was not the end of the story. In each case there were symptoms that did not fit the MS picture. And every one of the patients had tested positive for antiphospholipid antibodies. Hence their referral to Dr. Hughes.

As the patients' files were reviewed, the facts began to fit together like a jigsaw puzzle. Besides the neurological symptoms, a number of the women had suffered miscarriage, some had severe migraines, and others had arthritis. A majority showed white spots on their MRI scans, but that did not necessarily mean they had MS. Most important of all, though, was the positive blood test for antiphospholipid antibodies.

Staggering as it might sound, it transpired that *not one* of these twenty-seven women had MS; rather, they *all* were suffering from Hughes syndrome. This particular group was not merely a quirk. Since this report was published, an increasing number of patients have had a similar story to tell. The upshot is that Dr. Hughes believes blood tests for APS should be carried out in cases where the diagnosis of MS is unclear.

Patients' Stories

✱ Sally Evans

Among nonmedical people the general opinion is that doctors look after their own. If one of their fraternity becomes ill, she or he is fast-tracked through the health-care-system minefield and receives first-class treatment. The case of Dr. Sally Evans shows that this assumption is not always true.

Despite her status as a medical doctor, it took Sally seven years to get the right diagnosis. In that time she suffered terrible symptoms that inflicted permanent damage on her nervous system. At the age of forty she has to come to terms with the fact that part of her face will always be numb, that she is virtually blind in her right eye, that she has some problems with her left eye, and that she is incontinent. In the year 2000, she had to give up her job in a busy medical practice.

"I felt very unhappy for those seven years," she says. "I was constantly worrying about what was wrong with me. I found it desperately frustrating not to have a diagnosis. I began to think I was going mad. I started to think that I might be imagining my vertigo, the optic neuritis, or that I couldn't feel anything on my face. I underwent so many costly medical tests, and they showed nothing."

Because Sally had pushed for a second opinion, she was seeing two neurologists. She had been told she had multiple sclerosis. "I will never forget that moment," she recalls. "The doctor shook my hand, told me I had MS, and simply said good-bye. And that was it; there was nothing he could do, so I was shown the door."

Fortunately, Sally's other neurologist was not convinced. Her MRI scan showed no lesions or white blobs, and he felt her symptoms did not follow the pattern of MS. Furthermore, Sally's blood test for antiphospholipid antibodies was very, very high. At this point Sally had not heard of Hughes syndrome, nor had any of her medical contemporaries. Luckily her neurologist did know of the disorder, and she was referred to another specialist. Tests confirmed that she was suffering from APS rather than MS. She was put on warfarin and began to monitor her own INR (internationally normalized ratio; see more about monitoring one's own INR in Jeremiah's story, below). But a lot of damage had already been done; perhaps the hardest of which to accept was the loss of sight in one eye.

"I will never be able to practice medicine in the future," Sally says. "I persevered for a few years, but it just became too difficult. Imagine working in a doctor's office when you are incontinent, or when you cannot see properly. Most of the nerve damage will never improve. The numbness in my face is like having permanent dental anesthesia. When I eat, I dribble on one side; my smile is crooked; and when I talk to someone, I feel as though half my face is frozen. It makes you feel impersonal and detached.

"I am not bitter or angry that it took seven years to get a diagnosis. I know it might seem odd that it took so long even though I'm a doctor, but then perhaps it was because of my profession that I was more likely to ignore my symptoms. I would dismiss things and tell myself I was being a bit of a hypochondriac. I was less outspoken about what was going on, so I am partly responsible.

"One thing I do feel strongly about after being wrongly told I had MS is that doctors should not give a patient a diagnosis until they are absolutely sure about it. To be told you have a degenerative disease and then that you don't, and then to be told you have something else unpleasant is a terrible psychological shock."

✳ *Jeremiah Johnston-Sheehan*

Jeremiah is a talented architect. Now in his early forties, he has always taken care of his health. He watches his diet and gets regular exercise. One of his favorite pastimes is hiking in the hills. So the onset of an incurable illness was particularly hard on him. It was while he was walking in the Highlands of Scotland that he first noticed the change in his health. He would suddenly feel utterly exhausted, a paralyzing fatigue that made it hard for him even to get back to his car. He knew something was wrong and thought it might be linked to the asthma he had endured for many years.

Gradually, other symptoms developed. "I started having double vision, the beginnings of optic neuritis (inflammation of the optic nerve where it enters the eye)," he says. "Then I began to trip and to have problems with my balance. I had something called 'drop foot,' where I couldn't lift my toes, so I would fall over them. I was getting badly bruised; at one point I ended up in the ER with dislocated ribs and gashes. I looked as though I had been in a war. The doctors described me as 'a medical chaosity.'"

He was given an MRI scan. When the results came back, his neurologist asked him if he wanted the "good news" or the "bad news" first. Jeremiah's heart sank, but he went along with the game no matter how inappropriate. He wanted to hear the good news first. Relief came with the news that he did not have a brain tumor. But that optimistic moment was immediately crushed by the bad news. There were white markers on the scan. The diagnosis was probable secondary progressive MS.

"At one point I was admitted to St. Thomas' Hospital," he recalls. "I was surrounded by people with advanced-stage MS. I was sitting there looking around wondering if I shared their fate. The condition of these people was not something you see in an ER or anywhere else. There I was, at forty-two, seeing what might be around the corner for me. All I wanted to do was get on with my work, but it wasn't going to be that simple."

Of all the tests carried out on Jeremiah, there existed one blood result that didn't fit. He had antiphospholipid antibodies. "My neurologist didn't think it was significant, but he still felt the proper thing was to check it out by referring me to another specialist," Jeremiah says. "I had never heard of Hughes syndrome, so when I got home, I hit the Internet and within four hours I knew enough to understand that having this and not MS would definitely be 'good' news. Trouble was, they couldn't do a repeat blood test for months. It was Christmas, and my appointment wasn't until the following summer.

"I forced the neurologist to give me some odds: MS versus APS. He said there was an 85 percent chance I had MS and a 15 percent chance it was something else. At that point I was resigned to the fact that the only way for me to survive was to carry on as if it were MS. If I were wrong, well, so much the better; if not, I would have done what I could."

Jeremiah knew that beta-interferon was the only drug that seemed to slow down the progress of MS, and the earlier treatment began the better. The drawback was that Great Britain's National Health System would not pay for it. So he and his wife decided to fund the treatment themselves. It cost more than a thousand dollars a month, a lot of money to spend when extended over thirty years or more. Still, he says, "I had been through two years of feeling very unwell, months of tests, and then dealing with the news that I most likely had MS. I elected to start on the beta-interferon partly for the benefit of my wife and family. I felt I had to show them that I was doing something."

Jeremiah had been referred to a consultant rheumatologist and specialist in autoimmune diseases, Dr. David D'Cruz, at St. Thomas' Hospital. Blood tests were run again to see if the antibody was still present. Jeremiah had to wait for the results. He says it was the longest two weeks of his life. "When Dr. D'Cruz called me back and said, 'In my opinion you do not have MS; you have something called antiphospholipid syndrome,' I was overjoyed. I had read so much about sticky blood that I knew exactly what he was saying. It was such incredibly good news and a tremendous relief."

Once treatment with warfarin began, Jeremiah's symptoms started to disappear. "The medication kicked in very quickly," he says. "The tingling feeling in my fingers and toes went away, as did the double vision. In a matter of days I no longer needed the walking stick, and the fatigue started to dissipate."

The key to controlling the symptoms of APS is to maintain a delicate balance, to keep an eye on how thin or thick the blood is. Jeremiah does this by using a self-test kit, which he bought for about $450 and uses at home. It measures the blood's INR (internationally normalized ratio), which compares the thickness of the patient's blood with what you would expect to find in normal blood. The higher the ratio, the thinner the blood. Jeremiah feels well when his INR measures 3 to 4. Vigilance is crucial. He says, "If I have been under great stress—for instance, like when I was laid off at the end of 2001—then my condition begins to deteriorate. My INR drops, and with that the tingling, fatigue, mobility problems, and so on start to return. I test myself and see that I need to increase the warfarin. And so far this system works for me.

"Having had to live with the fear that I had MS was very traumatic, and because of that I do find it harder these days to cope with stress. But I also think that I had a chance to start over again, thanks to the team at St. Thomas', where they are inquisitive and challenge things. They ask questions and get answers, which is good news for people like me."

✳ ✳ ✳

Whatever doctor or clinic you work with, those last comments of Jeremiah's can be applied universally: What matters is that your medical team keep working with you to find answers, especially when tests and other investigations yield something besides the expected results.

Chapter 7

The Brain

Few things can be more frightening than realizing you are losing your memory, speech, and vision. To open your mouth and splutter out the wrong words, or to struggle to remember events that happened moments before are devastating symptoms. People with early Alzheimer's disease experience this deterioration, but it can also be a sign that antiphospholipid antibodies might be present. If that is the case, then the news is relatively good; it means rather than slipping into degenerative Alzheimer's disease, for which there is no cure and few treatments, you have APS and can be treated, often with highly effective results.

APS-Related "Brain Drain"

Graham Hughes has observed that a considerable number of patients come to him complaining of having a "foggy head." They recount how their self-esteem is damaged because friends or work colleagues who are used to their being on the ball notice the change and tease them about being slow or dim-witted. With these symptoms, if the problem is APS, the results of treatment are often dramatic. Patients talk of the fog lifting and of seeing things clearly again; they speak of their enormous relief at getting their speech and memory back.

Dr. Hughes believes this aspect of antiphospholipid syndrome must be examined more closely. He says, "Research to date is limited, but I feel certain that in time this syndrome will become widely recognized by psychologists and psychiatrists for patients with a variety of neurological disorders."

Besides "brain drain," Hughes syndrome can also cause major neurological disturbances, such as those described in the preceding chapter as mimicking the symptoms of multiple sclerosis. Dr. Hughes explains the impact of sticky blood on the brain by making an analogy with a car. When the mixture of fuel is too rich, the engine begins to stutter and stops working properly. One patient described these symptoms to me as being like a computer that has a virus and begins, out of the user's control, to do odd things.

Physiologically, what happens to a brain affected by APS? Clots, which appear as white blobs on an MRI scan, impair the normal functioning of the brain. Sufferers of these clots might have mini-strokes known as TIAs (transient ischemic attacks). If the TIA is a minor one, then the damage will be negligible; the patient might even fail to notice anything wrong. It is a different story if the individual suffers a series of TIAs; this scenario can cause permanent damage to the brain, affecting such areas as memory, speech, and vision.

Patients' Stories

✳ *Barbara Osborn*

Barbara Osborn thought she was going to die. In a matter of weeks the former flight attendant was transformed from a healthy, energetic mother of two into someone who was unable to walk and in constant need of help from others. She was consigned to a wheelchair, attacked by muscle spasms that were so violent she lost control of her body. Devastated by the mystery illness, she contemplated suicide. Barbara, who was thirty-eight at the time and lived with her husband and children, had been preparing to go back to work. But things didn't work out as she'd planned. She says, "The first thing I noticed was that my legs felt heavy when I was running up stairs—I was the kind of person who was always rushing everywhere. The heaviness would come and go, and I didn't think much of it. But then it became more frequent, and I thought I had better see my doctor."

She was referred to a neurologist, but in the following months her condition deteriorated. Her legs would suddenly give way under her, and she found it difficult to get out of bed without help. Worst of all, she didn't know what was wrong, as she hadn't received a diagnosis. Barbara and her doctors thought she had multiple sclerosis. "They took me in for tests," she recalls, "and I spent ten days in a hospital ward with people who had MS, some of whom were in the advanced stages of the disease. It was very grim and I was so frightened, watching these people dying and thinking that I would soon be just as sick as they were. I had got it into my head that this was what I had. And although the tests didn't confirm I had MS, the doctors said it was still possible I did have it."

Barbara's condition worsened. She became so unwell and unable to control her body that she could no longer walk. She says, "The spasms were like having an electric current shooting through my body and lifting my feet off the ground. On one occasion a spasm was so strong that it threw me backwards onto the coffee table, splitting my head open. I had to be rushed to the hospital.

"At one point I felt terribly low, because I believed I was becoming such a burden on my husband and children. It was then that I understood why people commit suicide. I thought in a cold, logical way about it as the only thing I could do to relieve the suffering I had brought upon my family." But Barbara struggled on against the illness. The frustrating thing was that despite endless tests, she still didn't know what was wrong.

Then there was a breakthrough. Something abnormal showed up in a blood test and Barbara was referred to a rheumatologist. It was suggested that she might have lupus. She says, "I had never heard of lupus, and the doctor was so vague in explaining it that I thought I must have both it *and* MS. My friends went to local libraries and read about the condition. The books were pretty old and painted a bleak picture. My friends all thought I was on my way out. There was so little information available about lupus even six years ago.

"Then a friend found the name of Dr. Graham Hughes, and I insisted on seeing him. One of the first things he said to me was, 'I bet they've told you that you have MS. Well, we will see about that.'"

Dr. Hughes says Barbara's case was the worst he had seen. He was certain that she did not have MS. He says, "Barbara was suffering from lupus, but I also felt that she had the classic symptoms of antiphospholipid syndrome."

After months of suffering, an inexpensive blood test was all that was needed to confirm that Barbara did not have MS, but rather Hughes syndrome, as well as lupus. Once she was treated with a blood thinner, her recovery was staggering. Within forty-eight hours the spasms were gone. "The change was so dramatic after I started taking warfarin," she says. "The spasms stopped and things started to improve within days. I could hardly believe it. I could get myself out of bed, and I was out of the wheelchair pretty quickly. Then I walked with the help of canes."

The wheelchair and canes are now long gone. Barbara shows little outward sign of the trauma she went through. Tall and slim, she walks unaided and is every bit as energetic as she was when the illness struck six years ago. She is still on medication and has her own blood-test machine to monitor her INR levels. She says she can tell when she is becoming ill again because her speech becomes muddled.

Barbara has dedicated her time to working for the charity that helps fund the lupus unit at St. Thomas' Hospital. She is also a key figure in the Hughes Syndrome Foundation.

✳ Jon Barber

When I phoned Jon Barber, he cheerfully told me that the moment he put down the phone he wouldn't remember one word of our conversation. The damage to his brain from repeated TIAs and strokes means he has virtually no short-term memory. "I don't have any friends these days," he says, "because I can't remember anyone. I know those who have made it to the long-term part of my memory, but all the rest is a blank." Jon, a former engineer, puts a brave and jovial veneer on how badly Hughes syndrome has affected him and those around him.

It was while driving his child's carpool that his life changed forever. "I was forty-one when it all began to happen," he says. "I was driving my eleven-year-old daughter to school. During the journey we had a heated argument about her not doing homework and missing school. I was driving back home when I got this incredible pain in my chest. I thought, 'Here we go, I am having a heart attack.' I went to the hospital and had a second episode while they were examining me. They did a number of tests but could find nothing wrong with my heart. They said I had suffered two massive angina attacks. They sent me to another hospital to have more tests. The results were clear, and the specialist said he hoped his heart was as strong as mine when he got to my age. He said I had the heart of a sixteen-year-old.

"A few months later I had another violent episode. Once again the doctors found nothing. They told me that none of the right enzymes were present in the blood to show that there had been a heart attack. I saw a cardiologist, and he said he could find nothing wrong with me. I was given a regimen of tablets and that was it."

But Jon did not recover; in fact, his condition worsened. He was frustrated and depressed by the lack of a diagnosis. His work suffered and he lost his job. He endured a few more painful attacks and then started to lose his speech. "Early on there were certain words missing. One of the first to go was the word *chess*. My daughter was trying to describe the game to me, and I had no idea what she meant. I simply couldn't grasp what the word meant. I lost that particular word for a couple of months. Then it came back suddenly when we were watching a game show and the question was, 'What is the game that uses knights and castles?' I blurted out, 'Chess.'

"Then in August 1999, on the night of the lunar eclipse, I got a blind spot in my left eye. There was this huge white blob in my vision and an indescribable pain in the back of my head. I once had a tooth taken out without an anesthetic, and the pain beat that; the dental work was pleasant in comparison. The next day I went to the optician, and he said I should go to the hospital right away, because the damage he could see was consistent with a stroke. Instead, I made an appointment to see my own doctor the following day. I went home to think about what was happening to me. It was then I experienced another blind spot."

Jon was due to see the chief ophthalmologist at his local hospital when he had a massive stroke. He lost his voice and the sight in his left eye. "It happened while I was in bed," he recalls. "I had just woken up and I was almost blind and I couldn't speak. They did lots of tests—ultrasounds, CT scans, and MRI scans."

The tests confirmed that Jon had suffered a major stroke. There was also evidence of hundreds of TIAs. One area of the brain showed substantial damage. Jon says, "I am told I had between 250 and 350 TIAs, or mini-strokes. On the scans you can see that a chunk of my brain is missing on the frontal right side, the part that deals with memory."

Three weeks after he got home from the hospital, he was still virtually blind and had no voice. His ophthalmologist said there was no way the sight in his left eye would come back; it was also doubtful his voice would return.

Jon continues, "I am a Christian, and every year I volunteer for a special gathering called Spring Festival, where I work as a steward. I feared that this year I would not make it. Then I woke up at 4:00 A.M. one morning and I had a sure knowledge I would get my sight and my voice back. I knew I would be able to ride my motorcycle, a Honda GL700, down to the festival and work as a steward. It was my dearest wish.

"Each day after that there was an improvement in both my speech and sight. Oddly, and embarrassingly, the first words that came back to me were some Arabic swearwords I'd learned while I was in the Army. Within two weeks I was well on the road to recovery. My neurologist said he had never seen anything like it; he was shocked by how quickly I got my voice back. And that certainty in the early hours of the morning was right: I was able to go to the Spring Festival on my motorcycle, and I was well enough to be a steward."

But there was no miracle cure for Jon's overall condition, which still didn't have a name. He had been ill for some years and was desperate to know what was going on. He saw a neurologist who told him he might have antiphospholipid syndrome. Jon immediately searched on the Internet to find out more about the condition. He discovered he wasn't alone in suffering this terrible autoimmune disease. He linked up with other people who had endured the same symptoms and the same agonizing journey to get a diagnosis. It was on the Net that he also came across the name of a specialist, to whom he obtained a referral from his own doctor.

He says, "The specialist took one look at me and said I had the classic symptoms of Hughes syndrome. He put me on warfarin, and it is marvelous how well the drug works. Within weeks things had improved dramatically. I used to have TIAs all the time. I have had only two since I started taking warfarin in September 2001. Under normal circumstances I would have had a hundred of them by now. Bits of memory have come back, but other bits are lost forever. I find I sometimes think I know something, but when I search my brain for it, there is nothing but a black hole.

"At one point I was housebound for fear of having a TIA on the street, but these days I feel much more confident that I can go out without something happening to me. My wife and two children have more freedom now, because I don't need someone with me when I leave the house. I still suffer depression and a few other symptoms, but in general I have gotten my quality of life back.

"How would I describe living with APS? It is like driving along a highway in a thick fog. You can't see properly, no matter how you try, but then when you take the warfarin, the fog lifts and suddenly you can see clearly again. It is a blessed relief."

Chapter 8

The Heart

One of the most dangerous aspects of Hughes syndrome is the potential for clots to develop in the arteries, giving the disease access to the major organs, where serious damage can be done. Coronary thrombosis, defined as clotting in an artery that carries blood to the heart, is a leading cause of heart attack. Arterial clotting can also lead to painful angina attacks.

Not the Usual Suspects

Frustratingly, as we saw with Jon's case in the preceding chapter, if APS is the culprit, the usual tests for angina or coronary problems come up negative, and the individual might be sent away with a clean bill of health, when everyone, doctors included, knows that he or she has suffered a serious episode of some kind.

Current evidence shows that APS involvement in coronary problems is less common than it is in other health conditions, such as clots in the brain or miscarriage. Nevertheless, it is still a potential culprit that cardiologists should look at closely. Perhaps knowing that someone carries the antiphospholipid antibodies would help to determine the treatment he or she should receive during or after a heart attack. A different type of anticoagulant drug might provide better results for such individuals, or a more aggressive approach to treatment might be required.

For some Hughes syndrome sufferers, a heart attack occurs after years of struggling to find out what is wrong with their body, years of wondering why the myriad of symptoms don't add up but rather leave doctors shaking their heads, mystified by the patient's long list of health problems.

A Patient's Story

✱ *Kay Thackray*

Kay Thackray had a heart attack when she was thirty-seven years old. The event was not the beginning of her story; it was more the climax. Kay had suffered from migraines since she was fourteen. As she got older, she also suffered blurred and double vision, pins and needles, fatigue, and muscle pain, causing her doctors to suspect that she probably had MS. At one point she was diagnosed as having an overactive thyroid. As she was being treated for this condition, her general health deteriorated.

She says, "The most awful thing was my worsening eyesight. It was so irritating. I could no longer read comfortably, because the words jumped all over the page, and using the computer at work reduced me to tears of frustration. I couldn't hold a newspaper up, as my arms were like lead weights and ached continually."

Kay's memory started to fail. She would forget what she was talking about in the middle of a conversation. She recalls, "My memory became so poor it was like my mind was a thick fog and I had to wade through it to recall things. I would do something, and five minutes later I had no recollection of it at all.

"I kept a diary of my daily symptoms. By now they were so weird I was trying to convince myself they were real. One night, my fingers on one hand went numb one by one and then gradually came back one by one. Another time, my coordination was so poor I couldn't undo the buttons on a child's shirt at the swimming pool. I would show the diary to my doctor; he would read it and shake his head in puzzlement."

The day Kay had her heart attack she had been busy running errands in the morning; it was when she was on her way home that the pain began. "As I drove home I felt a pain in my chest like indigestion," she recalls. "It very quickly got a lot worse, and I knew I was having a heart attack. I felt strangely calm and drove to the local clinic. I parked the car and said good morning to an acquaintance on my way in. Once safe inside the clinic, I sunk to the floor in complete agony."

Kay's doctor thought she was an unlikely candidate for a heart attack, but the ECG confirmed Kay's fears. An ambulance took her to the hospital as an emergency patient. She was given a "clot buster"—a powerful drug to quickly break up a clot—and monitored closely for twenty-four hours in the cardiac unit. As she tells it, "They asked me if I wanted a clot buster, but my head was spinning from the painkiller I had been given. The doctor told me I needed the drug because I almost certainly had suffered a heart attack, but I remember his warning me that once I had been given it, I could bleed from absolutely anywhere in my body and they might not be able to stop it. For the first time, I was terrified, but I agreed to have it.

"As I lay there in bed with this drug dripping into me, I imagined I would bleed to death at any moment, but strangely my overall feeling was still one of calm. The whole experience was surreal, as though I were watching all this happen to someone else. The doctors and nurses say I was smiling the whole time. Perhaps it was the diamorphine.

"Once I was out of the CCU I received twice daily heparin injections and aspirin. On the second day, a lady came around with library books. I explained I couldn't see well enough to read, but she insisted I try one with large print. To get rid of her, I gave in and took one. To my amazement, I could read; my eyes were totally clear. It was a miracle! I read constantly after that for the sheer joy of it. I felt ecstatic and puzzled as to why this had happened, but whatever the reason I didn't care; the main thing was I could read again."

Kay recovered and was discharged. She felt better than she had for a year or more, as most of her symptoms had disappeared, although why they had was a mystery. Later that year, however, she suffered a full-blown angina attack. She underwent an angiogram, which shows whether the arteries are blocked, and got the all clear. "I had completely clear arteries around my heart," she says. "They told me they were wide enough to drive a bus through."

One of the tests she received was for anticardiolipin antibodies; the result was positive. Kay says she wasn't told about this at the time. She learned about it only later, while she was in the office of a hematologist and saw him write down the words *lupus anticoagulant*. She had never heard of it, but at last she had a name for the illness that was causing her symptoms.

Kay went onto the Internet and discovered that there were plenty of others out there like her. She read everything she could find about antiphospholipid syndrome and concluded she probably had the condition. She realized she should be on warfarin. She asked her primary-care physician to refer her to a specialist. While she was waiting for her appointment with the specialist, Kay again ended up in the hospital with unstable angina. This time, though, things were different. She was treated by a young doctor who knew about APS. She says, "He couldn't understand why I wasn't on warfarin. He said I had tested positive for the antibodies, and if a heart attack wasn't a major clotting incident, what was? I could have hugged him. I was slowly discovering that doctors who understand Hughes syndrome are like gold, a rare breed to be treasured."

Kay and her husband traveled to see the specialist. His diagnosis was exactly what she had expected. "The doctor said I had described the symptoms of antiphospholipid syndrome, and the best thing for me was to be on warfarin. He said if I had been taking it ten years ago, I would never have had a heart attack, and without it the risk of another blood clot in the next ten years was fifty/fifty. He also advised me the warfarin treatment should be continued for the rest of my life. If I did this, he said, I would be 'home and dry.' Those words were so uplifting. When life seems difficult, I often tell myself that I am 'home and dry.' It never fails to cheer me up."

Chapter 9

Lupus and APS

It was while he was working with lupus patients in the 1970s that Graham Hughes first noticed the tendency of blood to clot too quickly in some of his patients. His observation led to clinical tests and the discovery that antiphospholipid antibodies (APLA) were present in a large number of lupus patients and were strongly linked to thrombosis (clotting) in lupus. In some cases the link was so strong it was felt that the presence of the antibodies warranted recognition as a subgroup to lupus. Dr. Hughes also noted that pregnancies among lupus patients who lacked the antibody suffered a lower incidence of miscarriage.

An even greater discovery was just around the corner. In the early 1980s, Dr. Hughes and his team confirmed their belief that the antiphospholipid antibodies were also present in some individuals who did *not* have lupus. This meant that the antibodies were far more common in the wider population than they had first thought. The disease caused by the presence of these antibodies was named *primary antiphospholipid antibody syndrome*, or simply *antiphospholipid syndrome*, or APS. (When it is associated with lupus or a related disease, it is referred to as *secondary APS*.) The discovery received international acclaim, and in honor of the doctor behind this pioneering work, the illness was christened *Hughes syndrome*, the name by which it is most commonly known in the United Kingdom.

Basics about Lupus

What is lupus (which is technically known as *systemic lupus erythematosus*, or *SLE*)? It is an autoimmune disease that causes episodes of inflammation in joints, tendons, and other connective tissues, as well as in some organs. It mainly affects women; nine out of ten cases are female. It is most common among women of childbearing age, but men and children can have it as well. Although there is limited public awareness of the disease, it is estimated that in high-risk groups it can affect as many as one in every two hundred people and is more common than multiple sclerosis or leukemia. Symptoms include chronic fatigue, joint and muscle pains, blood abnormalities, skin rashes, migraine, depression, heart or kidney failure, neurological problems, and chest pain. No one knows what causes lupus, but it is thought that genetics plays a part. It is an incurable disease, and until recent years, life expectancy in those it attacked was poor. Now, with a new generation of treatments, the disease can be controlled, and a majority of sufferers live a relatively normal life between flare-ups.

Two Distinct Diseases

Without a doubt there is an overlap between lupus and Hughes syndrome. Tests show that as many as 20 percent of lupus patients carry the antiphospholipid antibodies. What isn't yet known is how many people suffer from Hughes syndrome alone. It could be as many as one in two hundred people in high-risk groups. Because the discovery of APS resulted from work with lupus patients, the majority of early cases that were studied linked the two diseases. In the past decade or so, as more people have been diagnosed with primary APS, that perception has changed. Still, it is going to take time to separate the two conditions in some people's minds.

In fact, these two autoimmune diseases are quite different from one another. Lupus primarily affects women, whereas Hughes syndrome is more evenly distributed between the sexes. Another important difference is that lupus sufferers can go on to develop

Hughes syndrome, but it is extremely rare that it happens the other way around. If you have APS, you are unlikely at a later date to develop lupus.

There is still a lot of confusion about the two conditions and their association, both within the medical field and among the general public. The confusion is felt acutely by many patients, some of whom have been told that they have lupus, and years later are told that they also have APS. It is a common chain of events, but a distressing one for people who must grasp the implications of not one but two complex diseases. These individuals have often endured years of illness; some joke that they've taken so many drugs they rattle like a pillbox. There is no quick fix in such cases. One of the best things a patient can do is to learn as much as possible about both conditions and be determined to fight them.

Patients' Stories

* Karen David

Karen David, from Jackson, Tennessee, has struggled with a lifetime of ill health. "As far back as I can remember, I have had aches and pains," she says. "I recall my mom taking me to the doctor, who told me I had growing pains. I was always anemic, and had colds, flu, and pneumonia at odd times during the year. I always had trouble with heavy bleeding during my periods and later when I underwent numerous surgeries to correct endometriosis. I would then go through spells of feeling fine, only to start with the pains and infections all over again."

As with the majority of patients in the Hughes syndrome "limbo," Karen's road to diagnosis proved tortuously long and difficult, affecting the major portion of her adult life. She finally got there only to discover that she didn't have one major illness, but two. Here, she tells the rest of her own story:

"In 1988, at twenty-three years old, I had my first pregnancy. It was very rough. I was sick the whole time and finally had an emergency cesarean section. Will was six weeks premature. He died the next day. His lungs had not developed, and he suffered heart and kidney failure. It was a tough time. My husband, Scott, and I were grieving, and then I began to get sick again. Over the next four years I suffered three miscarriages and two ectopic pregnancies. Finally, at twenty-seven, I had a hysterectomy.

"The next year, we adopted our son, Luke. I began to feel a bit better, but when Luke was one year old, all the trouble began again. I started running a fever every day. I had severe fatigue, achy joints, chest pain, and a terrible rash on my face and arms. In the mornings when I got up, I felt tired before I even left for work. I would be in tears by 9:00 A.M. I just couldn't go on.

"Finally, after seeing doctor after doctor, I was diagnosed with lupus in 1995. By this point I couldn't even walk due to the pain in my legs. The muscles and joints in my legs felt as though I had been standing on my feet for three straight months with concrete blocks attached. I had pneumonia every other month, my face was numb, and I had headaches. I don't think there was one body part that didn't hurt.

"The doctor said I had gone undiagnosed for nearly ten years. Even after starting the steroids, the immunosuppressives, and the other medications, I suffered daily. Finally I had to quit work as a dental assistant; I couldn't keep a normal routine. I was being admitted to the hospital every few months.

"My doctor sent me to Johns Hopkins Hospital in Baltimore. The specialist I saw there, Dr. Michelle Petri, diagnosed me with antiphospholipid syndrome. She was great; she started me on Coumadin (warfarin) and Plavix (clopidogrel, another blood thinner), as I had endured numerous TIAs, as well as DVTs and one PE (pulmonary embolus; an embolus is a blood clot that travels, in the case of pulmonary embolus, to the lungs). Since then, it has been difficult to keep my INR regulated (INR is a measure of the blood's thinness; see Chapter 12). When it falls below 3.0, I start to experience numbness in my face, left arm, and leg. I also suffer severe migraine, slurred speech, confusion, and memory problems.

"It is so frustrating to be taking the medications to control this disease, yet still suffering if my INR is not exactly where it should be. There is so little information available in the United States about this condition, and it is hard to get my doctor's attention focused on thinning the blood more to improve the symptoms. After months of confusion, pain, numbness, hospitalization, and feeling as if I were going crazy, I started my own research into APS.

"I found Dr. Graham Hughes and the Hughes Syndrome Foundation website. When I read the information provided there, it was like reading my whole life story. After you drive down a road that you've driven daily, only to realize you are lost, and after you look at yourself in the mirror, only to realize you don't recognize your own face, you become frightened. At that point, you are ready to do whatever you can to get help. One day my son, who was eight, said, 'Mom, you need to have your brain rewinded.' It was then that I decided it was time to get more involved and do something. I made an appointment with Dr. Hughes.

"Now, I knew it would be costly to travel to London to see a doctor. Since the treatment was outside the United States, my health insurance wouldn't pay for it, and there was also the flight, hotel, food, etc. Still, I made the appointment and just went on faith that if it was meant for me to get to London and see Dr. Hughes, then God would provide a way. I set my appointment date and began to pray.

"God listened. All my friends from high school and college, as well as my family, held a fund-raiser to help me get the money I needed to see Dr. Hughes. The fund-raiser raised enough money to get me to London and back. I can't tell you what a gift it was to see Dr. Hughes and meet his staff and to know they truly care about their patients' well-being. The trip helped me to see that there is hope for all the many areas of health affected by lupus and Hughes syndrome. We still have to endure the terrible pain, the side effects of medication, and the ups and downs of feeling crazy, but help is out there.

"Dr. Hughes suggested a new treatment option to me, which included home testing and getting heparin injections. This has given me great hope, as it means I have a few more good days each month. Following this treatment keeps my blood more regulated and has made me feel better.

"I only wish there were more awareness of these conditions in the general community and among doctors, most of whom just don't understand. They can't understand how frustrating our daily life is. How we once could do normal things so easily, and then one minute we can't remember how to spell words correctly or even how to open a door. When most people come to a door, the automatic reflex is to turn the handle and open it. But when your brain is in a fog, you have to actually stop at the door and try to remember what it is you are supposed to do. It doesn't come to you automatically.

"Then you finally get the right treatment, your blood is regulated, the fog lifts, and once again you can open the door, just like everyone else."

✱ *Edwina Sewell*

When Edwina sent her story to me, she recommended I sit down with a large gin and tonic before I started reading. It was sound advice.

Despite repeated illnesses in her early years, Edwina qualified as a dental nurse; she trained as a civilian with the British Royal Army Dental Corps. Perhaps it was a childhood full of visits to doctors for a variety of ailments that made her feel at home with the smell of anesthetic and the sight of blood.

Edwina was a sickly baby, and her early years were dogged with strange illnesses. When she was eight, she developed herpes zoster, commonly known as shingles. Her physician had never seen it in one so young. As she tells it, "From the age of eight onward my health was never right. My mother was always being told I had growing pains, a bug, or a virus. Migraines were a frequent occurrence. My mother was told she was fussing too much. She knew something was wrong, but she was made to feel stupid and ignorant."

In her early teens, Edwina developed rheumatic fever following a severe throat infection. She was also treated for a heart murmur and a racing pulse. "I knew my health would never be normal again," she says. "I always seemed to be unwell. I couldn't keep up with my friends. I would come home from school exhausted and have to go to bed. My education suffered due to frequent migraines, which regularly made me absent from school. In 1973, I was bitten by an insect and reacted so badly I was taken to the ER. I had a rash that persisted for several weeks and seemed much worse after I had been exposed to the sun"—a common symptom of lupus.

Edwina's ill health persisted, including a bout of glandular fever and erratic menstrual periods. When she was twenty-two, in 1980, she developed severe pain in her eyes. At the same time, she began to lose control of her speech. She says, "I remember that I was taken to the local police station on one occasion and accused of being intoxicated. My speech was slurred, and I had enormous trouble trying to explain to the police that I was not drunk. I couldn't find the right words, and to make things worse, my balance was negatively affected. I recovered within an hour, leaving the police rather puzzled at my recovery and me very worried about my symptoms.

"In the summer of 1980, I saw a neurologist because of the persistent eye pain I had been having. I was also losing the sensation in my legs, and suffering severe migraines. He thought I had a brain tumor, but nothing showed up on the CT scan. There were further investigations, but they found nothing. No diagnosis was made, and I was told my symptoms were 'all in my head.' I swore I would never see the neurologist again. I decided to forget my health problems and get on with my life.

"My job took me to a new city where I helped to set up a new dental practice, so I was working long hours. I was very tired. I had a massive attack of herpes simplex, more commonly known as cold sores. This was to be the first of many such attacks that would trouble me for years to come. The virus made me very ill. It seemed to trigger the neurological problems again. It was so bad I could not work. I lost the job I loved and had to move back to my parents' house.

"In 1982, I underwent general anesthetic for a dental operation. I reacted badly, and a few weeks later I developed a secondary infection that failed to respond to heavy-duty antibiotics. I became very unwell, so I was admitted to the hospital. Overnight, I became weak down one side of my body. I also lost my vision in one eye. Once again I was referred to a neurologist."

Edwina was told she had multiple sclerosis. Later that year she was again admitted to the hospital and put on large doses of steroids. Her eyesight had become so bad that she was registered as partially sighted; she left the hospital in a wheelchair because she was too fatigued to walk. Over time the steroids seemed to help, and Edwina managed to return to work part-time, but the unpredictability of her condition—in particular the frequent migraines—forced her to retire in 1984.

"Over the next few years," she says, "my parents and I questioned the diagnosis of MS because I did not 'do' what the textbooks said I should. I was investigated for epilepsy, but the tests were negative. I developed frightening mood swings that hit me out of the blue. I had episodes of slurred speech, confusion, and weakness in my limbs. The doctors said these were common complications of MS. I was convinced I was imagining the symptoms.

"I continued to doubt the diagnosis; then one morning toward the end of 1988, I woke up to find that I was weak down the right side of my body. My right hand and arm were badly affected. A local doctor gave me a high-dose steroid injection, and the neurologist said the MS had 'relapsed.' But I realized I had suffered a peripheral nerve palsy in my arm, which MS does not cause, as it attacks only the central nervous system. I pointed this out to my doctor, who still insisted I had MS."

Edwina changed doctors, but got the same verdict: that she had MS.

She continues, "A few more years passed, and my life became intolerable. My health was deteriorating, but the doctors would not listen to me or my parents. It was now very obvious to me that my symptoms could not be caused by MS, but at the same time I began to doubt my own judgement. I started to think I should accept the diagnosis I had, but I knew in my heart it was wrong.

"In 1991, I noticed pain in my hip. It became impossible to walk, and I found myself in the ER undergoing tests. They found I had avascular necrosis (the death of localized tissue, in this case resulting in the crumbling of her hip joint). The orthopedic surgeon I saw questioned the diagnosis of MS but was overruled by my general practitioner and neurologist. No one even mentioned to me that the problem with my hip could have been caused by the prolonged use of steroids."

Over the next few years, Edwina retreated to her bedroom; she was virtually housebound. She was sick and disillusioned with a medical profession that couldn't, or wouldn't, find out what was really wrong with her.

In 1993, she developed swollen joints and was admitted to the hospital. Septic arthritis was diagnosed. It was treated with antibiotics, but she went on to suffer severe chest pains. Edwina's doctors discovered that she also had pleurisy (inflammation of the membrane that covers the lungs and lines the inside of the chest wall) and pericarditis (inflammation of the lining around the heart).

She says, "About this time, I had a very abnormal reaction to the sun. I was sitting in the garden one afternoon when I noticed a rash on my exposed parts. This started to form into very tiny blisters, and I started to swell up. An hour later I was very uncomfortable—and worried about my appearance. The next day I was due to see a specialist, who redirected me to the ER for emergency treatment. For the first time, lupus was mentioned. I had never heard of it.

"I underwent an MRI scan, which confirmed that I definitely *did not* have MS and never had had MS. I wanted an apology from the doctors who'd put me through absolute hell for the past ten years—I had been on an emotional roller coaster. And now I had no name for my symptoms. Although I never believed I had MS, at least I'd had a name. Now there was no label. What was I to say if people asked what was wrong with me?

"My consultant was certain I had lupus, but the tests seemed to prove him wrong. They did find I had a connective-tissue disease, of which I was told there were many.

"I spent the next three years with no diagnosis and no treatment. My health continued to deteriorate, and I hit an all-time low. Nobody seemed to understand how I needed a label for my symptoms. I needed a diagnosis. I needed to know what I was fighting."

Edwina was admitted to the hospital on a number of occasions. At one stage she was so ill she lost consciousness, and her parents were told to expect the worst. But she pulled through. The list of her symptoms was daunting:

- severe migraine

- vertigo

- fatigue

- chest/joint/muscle pain

- hair loss

- partial hearing loss

- memory loss

- confusion

- visual disturbances

- hearing voices

It was only by chance that Edwina finally got on the road to a diagnosis. While she was visiting her parents, who had moved away, she hurt her back. She saw an orthopedic surgeon, who heard her medical history and said she must have lupus. When she said her blood test for lupus was negative, he told her she could still have lupus.

She says, "I went home and visited the library, where I saw a copy of *The Lupus Book*, by Daniel Wallace. He stated in black and white that it was possible to misdiagnose MS for lupus, and that it was also possible to diagnose lupus even with a negative blood test. That same week, my mother and I saw Dr. Graham Hughes talking about lupus on television. Everything he said seemed to relate to me. We couldn't believe what we were hearing. I knew I had to get referred to Dr. Hughes.

"I saw him six months later. He diagnosed lupus, Sjögren's, and possible antiphospholipid syndrome. (Sjögren's syndrome is a chronic inflammatory condition characterized by excessive dryness of the eyes, mouth, and other mucous membranes.) He didn't hesitate, and above all, he understood how ill I felt and the fight I'd gone through to reach his door. The relief was absolutely overwhelming. I finally had a name for all my symptoms. They could all be explained, and for the first time they all made sense. I was not imagining my symptoms, and I certainly wasn't crazy."

But getting the treatment right took time. Edwina reacted badly to a number of the medications. The anti-inflammatory drug azathioprine caused liver problems. It also transpired that years without a diagnosis had taken their toll. "It was apparent that the great delay in obtaining the correct diagnosis had caused irreversible damage to my body," she says. "I have severe calcinosis (a deposit of calcium, in Edwina's case, in her muscles). This affected my mobility and has left me with a gait that must be seen to be believed. The calcinosis and prolonged use of steroids have also caused muscle wastage, which also affects my mobility.

"In 1998, I was put on methotrexate (an immunosuppressive drug). It made a vast difference in the joint pains and some of the other lupus symptoms. I was able to maintain a reasonable state of health if I stayed on low-dose steroids, Plaquenil (an antimalarial drug that has proven useful in treating lupus-related rash), methotrexate, and baby aspirin. However, I still found that my life was being controlled by the endless migraines, confusion, memory loss, visual disturbances, and a weird brain 'fog' that made me lose track of time.

"It was decided in September 2001 that I should start taking warfarin, and I must say I have never looked back. My life has improved so much that I can now say I have a life—not just an existence. Within weeks of starting this treatment, I was able to shower and dress every day for the first time in about twenty years. To any healthy individual this may sound crazy, but to me it was a huge achievement. Still, it has been difficult to maintain the correct INR. Without any doubt, if it drops below 3.5, all my symptoms return.

"I could not have considered writing this essay if I were not taking warfarin. I would have typed the wrong letters, I would have lacked the concentration, I would not even have gotten out of my bed if I had a migraine or brain fog. It hurts terribly when I look back and think about what could have been if I had received the correct diagnosis years ago. My health stopped me from getting married and having children. My career was cut short. My family has sacrificed so much to let me have some degree of independence. Financially, life is an endless struggle.

"I continue to take each day as it comes. I have to pace myself if I am to keep some control over the fatigue, which in hindsight is much better than it used to be. I have learned not to ignore symptoms, and I ask for help when I know I am heading for a flare. I can now cope with my mood swings much better, because I no longer have persistent migraines and confusion. If my mobility improved, it would be an added bonus. If the pleurisy and pericarditis disappeared permanently, it would be a double bonus.

"I find the ignorance about both lupus and Hughes syndrome appalling. I attend a local hospital anticoagulation clinic where they admitted they had never heard of antiphospholipid syndrome. I am one of the fortunate ones who has been diagnosed and treated. I hope my experiences will help others who are still striving for the correct diagnosis."

✳ ✳ ✳

The message of hope in these two stories is that neither Karen nor Edwina ever gave up in their search for improved health, despite perhaps being tempted to do so, and despite the daunting obstacles thrown into their paths by their debilitating symptoms. As both women attest, finally getting the right diagnosis, even though it confirmed that they had an incurable disease, brought them great relief. Read on for more about the struggle for a diagnosis—and about how you can help yourself in that struggle.

Chapter 10

The Fight for a Diagnosis

A frequent problem for APS sufferers is the difficulty they go through to get a diagnosis. Of all those I interviewed for this book, not one had a straightforward path to finding out what was wrong with them. Most often it was quite the opposite: They endured a terrible struggle to find answers and obtain the right treatment. A few did have the good fortune to come across more enlightened medics who kept up to speed with the latest news in medicine and thus knew what Hughes syndrome was. Sadly, at the present time, those doctors are few.

Many APS sufferers go through months or even years of uncertainty before they discover what the mystery illness is that has ruined their health. Most people I have spoken to talked of getting to the point where they feared they might be going mad or turning into a hypochondriac. In defense of the doctors, it is fair to say that APS affects individuals in many different ways, so no two cases are alike. This fact makes diagnosis very difficult.

Accessing the Help Available

I found it interesting that quite a few people discovered what was wrong with them by searching the Internet. Growing numbers of people meet in cyberspace and compare notes on APS. (For some of the websites that sponsor APS-related chat rooms or discussion groups, see Resources.) This is a phenomenon that has evolved without preconception or plan but through the sheer need of so many to know more. It is also quite telling that people are turning away from the doctors who don't know, and are finding answers for themselves from fellow sufferers.

In a case where someone has been diagnosed with lupus, it is slightly easier to expose the antiphospholipid antibodies; the patient already has a recognized autoimmune disease, so her or his blood will be tested regularly. However, the majority of APS sufferers start from square one, and that makes it harder to get a diagnosis. It is quite common for patients to have consulted with a variety of medical specialists over a period of many years, but still be in the dark about what is making them so ill. The diversity of symptoms confuses the picture and leaves doctors puzzled and unable to provide patients with the answers they need.

As we've seen, many of those who do find themselves in front of qualified specialists and who do get the proper diagnosis are the ones who employ a combination of determination and luck. They are the ones who shout the loudest. It often takes time, but they get there in the end. Still, APS is by many accounts relatively common. If Graham Hughes is right, it will soon eclipse other autoimmune diseases. So where are all the other sufferers of the disorder? A widely held fear is that those who are too ill to fight or who have difficulty "shouting loud" are being overlooked. Another concern is misdiagnosis. How many people diagnosed with MS actually have Hughes syndrome? What about those who have suffered terrible migraines for years, when the proper diagnosis of APS could have helped them find ways to deal with the pain? What about patients who have been told they have early dementia, yet do not? Or the women who keep losing babies through miscarriage? It is a disturbing thought that possibly thousands of individuals are struggling with terrible symptoms without knowing what is wrong, perhaps writing themselves off as hypochondriacs while gradually becoming more ill as the disease continues to attack them and to remain untreated. These people are not getting the help available.

Even though an inexpensive blood test exists and effective drugs are readily accessible, they suffer in silence. Perhaps the stories of those who were eventually heard will help show them the way.

Patients' Stories

✳ *Ann McFall*

Ann says she had a headache for eighteen years. It's hard to believe, but almost every day of her life after the birth of her son, she was plagued with various degrees of pain in her head. And the older she got, the worse it became. No matter what tests were carried out and which specialist she saw, they could find nothing wrong. The results were all negative. For Ann, the frustration turned into depression and the fear that she was imagining the symptoms.

She says, "Think what it would be like if as soon as you opened your eyes in the morning you got a pain all over your eyes like a terrible hangover, pain that made you feel so bad you had to run to the toilet to be sick. Worse still, what if no painkillers worked? That was what it was like for me for years, ever since my son was born in 1983. The only thing I could do was lie on the bed with a damp cloth over my eyes, but even then I couldn't sleep because of the pain. It was horrible. I think my poor husband must have gotten sick of my moaning about how bad my head felt. It made me so bad-tempered with everyone because I couldn't be myself."

Ann, who is thirty-nine, spent almost half her life trying to find out what was wrong in the hopes that she could stop the pain. She continues, "After my Ryan was born, I was quite sick, and no one knew why. I had headaches and joint pains. At one point they thought something was wrong with my liver. My skin started to go blotchy. I was in and out of the hospital for tests, but they all came back negative. In the end I felt I must be neurotic. I was convinced everyone thought I was a hypochondriac. However, my doctor was very concerned about me, and prescribed some special migraine medicine.

"In 1990, they did find something in my blood, at long last. At the time, they said it showed that I had rheumatism, but now I know it was more likely lupus. In any event, all of that was put to one side when I got pregnant.

"The pregnancy was a disaster. I lost my baby at six months. I kept telling the doctors that I didn't feel well and I knew there was something wrong. Tests had shown that my thyroid wasn't working, and my GP said they would keep a close eye on me. My water broke early, and we went to the hospital. The doctor there said they must get the baby out; he said they would give me a labor-inducing drug to make it quick, but it took twenty-four hours. The baby was dead. They lay it near me and then took it away. I was hysterical. I was beside myself.

"After that I was very ill. All my symptoms became a hundred times worse. They thought I had septicemia. I think it was after losing my baby that the lupus really kicked in. My GP at the time was brilliant. She did keep a close watch on me, and in the end she thought something strange was going on. When I was pregnant with my daughter in 1993, she got me a referral to a lupus pregnancy clinic. I was monitored closely. It was a difficult pregnancy, but my little girl, Ellie, is now eight, so something must have gone right."

After Ellie's birth, the headaches became even more ferocious, and Ann developed other symptoms. She had numbness in her fingers, toes, and parts of her face, a condition known as *peripheral neuropathy*. Her joints were swollen, and her skin was covered with rashes. She suffered chronic fatigue, as well as flulike symptoms, including a high temperature. She says, "My skin would get so bad I wouldn't leave the house. I would stay indoors and cry. If I did go out, young children would look at my skin and ask if I had cancer.

"In September 2000, I saw a specialist who did some more tests, which confirmed I had antiphospholipid syndrome as well as lupus. He put me on warfarin. It was so nice to talk to a doctor who understood what I had; he didn't make me feel that I was mad. He would ask me if I had a certain symptom, and when I said yes, he would calmly nod his head. It was great, because he knew what I was going through. I thought, 'Oh thank God, this is someone who believes me.'

"Within two weeks the headaches were gone; it was heaven. Suddenly it was a pleasure to get up in the morning. I didn't have the pain, and so I wasn't grumpy with the kids. I did, however, wonder if the pain would come back. Nowadays I still get the occasional headache, but nothing like what I used to suffer. The specialist said he suspected I had no quality of life because of the pain I was suffering, and he said the treatment would change that. He was right; I do now have a good quality of life, and I am grateful for each day that passes without a headache.

"I really hope and pray that people are made aware of both conditions—lupus and Hughes syndrome. I think there must be a lot of people out there who don't know they have these conditions. Before I knew what I had, at times I felt that I wanted to die. But once I knew what was wrong, I no longer felt like a freak. It was such a relief."

✳ *Kate Welch*

Young people never expect to become ill, so Kate Welch was stunned when she ended up in the hospital with a clot in her right calf at the age of thirty-two. A successful systems analyst in Chicago, Kate had never been seriously unwell. She had just gotten married and was a highly motivated career woman.

As she tells it, "Three months before the clot happened, I had been to see a doctor because I just didn't feel right. I was under a lot of stress. At work there was a company merger, and I was newly married. My heart would race and then beat strangely. At times I was totally exhausted for no reason, and my vision started to go. I generally felt light-headed and dizzy. On top of all that, I couldn't seem to concentrate on things the way I used to.

"I didn't think the outside events in my life should have made me feel so bad. I have always been a high-energy, career-motivated, 'take-on-the-world' kind of person. So after doing some tests, including heart imaging, lung scan, and basic blood exams, my doctor determined that I probably had costochondritis, which is an inflammation of the cartilage between the ribs. He told me to take it easy and said the rib pain would probably stop soon. It was only later that I found out costochondritis is an autoimmune response.

"Then, three months later, in April 2000, I was checked into the hospital with the clot. I felt that my internist was totally incompetent and failed to run the right tests. It took three months to find this out, because both she and the hospital lost my records. When I asked about support stockings, she said I didn't need them, and she wanted to take me off Coumadin (warfarin) after only three months. When I said I wanted to stay on the drug longer, she said, 'What will people think?'—as if that mattered. In any case, I searched the Internet and learned so much. I was able to find out what tests were supposed to be run, and in August I found another doctor who agreed to run some of the right tests. And *voilà*! I was positive for anticardiolipin antibodies.

"My current doctor is much better. He is also a hematologist, so he understands a lot more about the problem. But he still does not seem to associate the APS with any of my 'stress' symptoms. Whenever I would say I just didn't feel right, he would dismiss it as stress. It wasn't until I found the Forum, a website on the Internet (http://forums.delphiforums.com/apsantibody/messages), and read about other people's symptoms and day-to-day lives with the disease that I finally understood why I was feeling strange. Looking back, I can see that the 'stress' symptoms were actually the beginnings of the syndrome. I also now know that the symptoms are not necessarily all because of stress, and that I am not going crazy or just being a hypochondriac! It is a very real part of the disease and I believe it is one of the things doctors know least about.

"As for what impact APS has had on my life, you could say it has rocked my world. I am so lucky to have an understanding spouse and supportive parents, but life as I knew it will never be the same. I used to be full of life, outgoing, popular—nothing could stand in my way and I loved my life. I am now anxious, afraid, lonely, my self-confidence waxes and wanes, and I have gained twenty-five pounds. Between the employment uncertainty and my health uncertainty, I have not been able to finish my master's degree, and I fear I may never get it done. I am also registered to take the PE (professional engineer's) exam, but I cannot fathom being able to work full-time while I study. In the past, this would not have phased me. I completed my master's coursework while working full-time and enjoying a very active social life. Now I am just exhausted all the time, and I have little enthusiasm for most things. The exhaustion is the hardest for me to get used to since I was never tired like this before. However, I do consider myself lucky as far as my work goes. I am currently able to go to the doctor whenever I need to, and I can run out for INR blood tests easily. I feel that I am very lucky in that way; I am sure most people do not have such flexible and understanding bosses.

"Managing the disease once you are diagnosed becomes a major part of life. This involves getting regular blood tests, changing the diet, no drinking. Then there's all the time spent looking for answers from different doctors and on the Internet, trying to connect with other people who feel as you do, and trying to make some sense of why this happened when you were perfectly healthy before.

"Another huge impact has been the issue of having children. Pregnancy is very uncertain and requires shots, and no one can predict the impact of the disease on the fetus during pregnancy. Then there's the increased risk for the mother of developing another life-threatening clot. My biggest concern is with the hereditary considerations of the disease. The current literature says it is not genetic, but it 'tends to run in families.' So my husband and I were worried about whether we should risk having children of our own; we thought it might be better to adopt. It was so depressing for me; I felt I couldn't bear the thought of another human being going through this because of my selfishness.

"We looked closely at our family histories. Certainly autoimmune conditions did not seem to run in my family, although my mother did have a clot a few days after I was born. I was born via cesarean section, and she was forty-two years old at the time. Although she is factor V Leiden positive, she has never been on anticoagulant therapy (except for the first six months after her clot) and has not had any problems since. Now she is a very healthy seventy-four-year-old. Luckily, she did not pass the factor V Leiden gene on to me." Factor V Leiden is a variant form of factor V, a normal substance in the blood that aids with clotting. Individuals who have this variant are more likely to develop blood clots than those without it.

Kate continues, "We also went to the University of Chicago Hospital for a genetic-counseling session. We spoke with the head of the department. She felt that APS was not a hereditary condition, and that I should go ahead and have children and not worry about it. My primary-care doctor and my gynecologist also did not see any reason to avoid having children. I am still concerned, but we traced the family history and there really does not seem to be any evidence of Hughes syndrome or any other autoimmune problems. So we are going to proceed with trying to have one or two children of our own. I am dreading the shots, and I am trying to get myself into the best physical condition I can before we start down the pregnancy path.

"My condition is stable. I wear full-height compression stockings, and I get my INR checked once a month. I am learning to accept my new life. I am trying to exercise regularly and lose some weight, but it's really hard because I'm so tired most of the time. Still, I will get there in the end."

✻ *Carole Judge*

Fifty-four-year-old Carole has strong feelings about the current lack of awareness regarding Hughes syndrome. After what she and many others have been through, Carole believes a media campaign should be conducted on television, radio, and in the press to let people know about the disorder. She feels that if more of the public and more doctors knew of the condition, there would be a lot less unnecessary suffering.

"I used to work as a catering manager at a college," she says, "but I had to retire two years ago because of ill health. I have several conditions. They include Raynaud's, which I have had since I was a child; fibromyalgia, which was diagnosed five years ago; lupus; Sjögren's; and antiphospholipid syndrome, discovered just recently." Raynaud's phenomenon is a condition in which small arteries, usually in the extremities, go into spasm, causing the skin to turn pale or discolored. Fibromyalgia is an illness characterized by achy pain and stiffness in the muscles, tendons, and ligaments.

Carole continues, "In 1991, I was taken ill while on vacation. I had an allergic reaction to the sun, and I also suffered a gastric viral attack. I was having lots of different health difficulties: kidney problems, irritable bowel symptoms, joint pains, fatigue, skin rashes, insomnia. I gained weight, although my eating habits had not changed. I developed memory problems; it was like being dyslexic with words and numbers. I would start to write the next word before I had finished the one I was on. I found I could not remember names of people I had worked with for a long time, or procedures I had followed for many years. Now I have a number of symptoms: TIAs (mini-strokes); patches of skin that are red and get larger, sometimes going septic; red spots on my fingers; and deterioration of my kidney function.

"I was told by two specialists to see someone else. I was told by another specialist that it was all in my mind and to 'go home and have some aromatherapy.' Because of what that doctor wrote on my hospital notes, my general practitioner wanted to put me on tranquilizers and refused to believe I was ill. So I changed GPs. The one doctor's notes were still on my records, so when I was admitted into the hospital in 2001 and started having TIAs, the specialist I was under did not believe me and would not treat me. She, too, told me to see someone else. If it were not for my family, I would have thought my symptoms were in my imagination. I got angry that nobody seemed to help me or want to help me.

"The turning point was finding Dr. Hughes—it's that simple. He listened to me, he asked questions, and he believed me. He diagnosed lupus, Sjögren's, and APS. The relief I felt was tremendous. He restored my faith in doctors.

"We need to educate the medical profession in how to listen to their patients. My new and excellent GP told me that some doctors will not admit they have no idea what is wrong with someone, so they tell the patient it is their fault or all in their mind. I would like to see people talking about APS on the television, hear them on the radio, and see posters in all doctor's offices.

"I would advise any person who has an illness but can't get a diagnosis for it to keep on fighting. See different doctors, make a noise, and stand up for yourself. Remember that many doctors do not want to take on complicated cases."

Depression

A worrisome number of patients I spoke to have had an extremely difficult struggle to get a diagnosis because doctors really did think their symptoms were all in their minds. These individuals were written off as neurotics or hypochondriacs. In some cases they found themselves treated for depression for many years, while the APS symptoms got worse. It is tough to stand up to doctors and say you are not depressed, or that you are depressed but it's because of your illness. When you are unwell, it is hard to find extra energy to fight, but with such an unfamiliar condition as Hughes syndrome it is when you are the most ill that you need strength to take on the medical establishment. Those who give up too easily could be consigning themselves to years of being prescribed antidepressants—and a worsening physical condition.

* Judi Page

For many years Judi Page was treated for depression. She complained of a wide variety of symptoms, but none of them were treated as part of a whole picture until recent years.

"I have not been 100 percent fit since having glandular fever when I was sixteen," she reports. "I got tired easily and I had no stamina. But that might have been due to the Sjögren's syndrome, which I also suffer from; it was diagnosed in 2001, at the same time as the APS. It seems sticky blood is often accompanied by various other complaints.

"The problems got worse after I had pneumonia just over fourteen years ago. I started suffering from migraine, eczema, IBS (irritable bowel syndrome), depression, and fatigue. For many years doctors put it all down to depression. Then about two years ago, the migraines and the IBS got much worse. Last summer I endured headaches every day, many of them incapacitating. I also fell over a few times for no apparent reason; at one point I fell down a flight of stairs.

"The doctors investigated the migraines and the falls; their tests revealed I had something wrong with my heart. I was diagnosed with angina, and the falls were labeled as resulting from vasovagal syncope (fainting).

"As you can see from the more than fourteen years it took to find out what I was suffering from, I had extreme difficulty getting a diagnosis of APS, possibly because the symptoms were put down to depression. Even after things got really bad a year ago, the rheumatologist missed it. He diagnosed Sjögren's and tested me for lupus; the result was negative. He missed the antiphospholipid syndrome, despite the fact that I have been told more recently it should have been obvious I was suffering from this condition.

"I did some of my own research on the Internet about lupus and Hughes syndrome. I decided I would see a specialist as a private patient. I underwent a blood test for the antibodies, and it came back normal. As a result, my general practitioner wasn't convinced I had APS and once again said my problems were due to depression. Then I had an MRI brain scan, which showed two small abnormalities, but even that was ignored.

"I found another specialist. Luckily, he didn't believe the blood-test result from my local hospital, so he retested me. My level of antiphospholipid antibodies was high. It is a good thing I am persistent. I nearly gave up many times, because no one, apart from a couple of friends, believed me. At long last I got a diagnosis of APS in November 2001.

"I would say to others with this condition that they must remember that their regular doctor probably won't have had a patient with this illness before. So you must inform yourself as much as you can to back yourself up and help you fight for a referral to a specialist who is experienced in this field."

A Note to North American Readers

You may have noticed that several of the individuals whose stories are told in these pages have found understanding and relief only after consulting with Dr. Hughes in London. It is true that antiphospholipid syndrome seems to be somewhat better known in the United Kingdom than it is in North America, in large part thanks to the efforts of Hughes and his team. Due to this greater awareness among the British medical community, APS patients in the United Kingdom can usually get the necessary referral to St. Thomas' Hospital to consult with the specialists there. But what if, as is the case for the vast majority of North American APS patients, you aren't in a position to travel to England to receive specialized medical treatment? How can you help yourself?

It pays to realize that for the time being the need to be proactive seems to apply even more to APS patients who live in North America. They often find themselves in the position of having to educate not only themselves but also their health-care providers about the illness. Many tell stories of mentioning antiphospholipid syndrome to their physician, and finding that the doctor has never heard of it. Take inspiration from the case studies in this book, and decide to do whatever is required to get the proper diagnosis and treatment for your condition. Resolve to follow the tips listed in Chapter 1 for how to be a proactive patient. Show your health-care providers this book and any other literature you obtain about Hughes syndrome. By doing so, you'll be helping yourself as well as spreading the word about the disorder, an action that will benefit other APS patients.

No matter where he or she lives, good news does exist for the Hughes syndrome sufferer who persists in fighting to get a diagnosis. This good news is that positive options for managing the illness do exist, usually in the form of effective, safe, and relatively inexpensive drug treatment. But be aware that for many, these rewards come only as a result of educating oneself about the disease and all of its ramifications, asserting oneself with the medical community, and—perhaps most important—refusing to give up.

Chapter 11

Catastrophic Antiphospholipid Syndrome

The most frightening manifestation of APS is a serious condition with the ominous-sounding name of *catastrophic antiphospholipid syndrome*, sometimes abbreviated as CAPS. Fortunately, the disorder is extremely rare, but when it does happen, the impact on the body is devastating. Without immediate treatment it can kill.

A Medical Emergency

The condition occurs when a person who has the antiphospholipid antibodies (APLA) suddenly develops clots all over his or her body. In the few cases of CAPS that are documented, it is not uncommon for the patient to have been generally healthy before the attack; they might not even know they carry the antibody. The clots appear throughout the whole body and can cut off the blood supply to a few or all vital organs, potentially disabling many bodily systems. This is a full-blown medical emergency; treatment must be speedy and aggressive to save the patient's life.

No one knows what causes this terrible disorder; however, in some patients it appears to be triggered by an infection, such as a virus or sore throat. Another extremely rare cause is stopping anticoagulant drug treatment in a Hughes syndrome patient.

A Patient's Story

* Alan Varney

Alan Varney, an engineer, moved across the country when he was in his early fifties. The move left him tired and breathless, which puzzled him, as he was otherwise energetic and felt well. He had been quite healthy most of his life, other than suffering some annoying ulcers on both legs that needed pressure dressings. But this didn't bother him. He was more concerned that three months after the move he was still breathless.

"My doctor thought I was asthmatic," Alan says. "He gave me an inhaler and told me to see him again in a week. But I was back before the week was up because I felt worse. I was still going to work, which involved a lot of driving. During one trip I had a sharp pain in the right side of my chest. I told no one, but I must have looked unwell, because one of my colleagues insisted on driving me home. To be honest, I knew I was unable to drive at that stage."

Alan's recollections from this point on are hazy, so his wife, Marian Varney, tells the rest of the story.

Marian recalls, "Alan had a very bad night. He was vomiting and just wasn't himself. He lost his coordination and started rambling. I told him I should call an ambulance, but he wouldn't have it. In the morning he couldn't walk properly. I'm not sure how I got him to the doctor's office. Once we were there, our family doctor thought the problem might be neurological and got him a bed at the hospital. No one would confirm he had suffered a stroke, but that was what we both thought. The nurse, however, pointed out that a stroke normally affects only one side of the body, whereas Alan was having problems with coordination on both sides."

Alan's doctors didn't know what had made him so ill. After a week they said he could go home for the weekend, but they changed their minds when they found a clot on his lung. Over the next twelve days, Alan's feet grew darker in color, a symptom that came and went. Meanwhile, he underwent daily blood tests and was obviously deteriorating.

"At one point," Marian says, "I came into the ward and there were three consultants gathered around Alan's bed. I knew there must be something terribly wrong. They told me they had found something abnormal in his blood. It was called antiphospholipid antibody. I just couldn't get my head around that term. I made them repeat it time and again, and then I got them to spell it out so I could write it down. I had also heard that Alan might have lupus. It was by sheer luck that I had noticed lots of leaflets about lupus in the waiting room. I had heard of that disease but had no idea what it was. On the leaflet was the address for a lupus organization. I contacted it, and the staff of the organization sent more information about antiphospholipid syndrome. When I showed the material to the nurses on Alan's floor, they asked for a copy, because they had never heard of APS before."

Marian's feeling of foreboding when she saw the team of consultants at her husband's bedside was not misplaced. Alan's legs had become gangrenous, and although no one really knew what was wrong with him, the decision was made that the legs had to be removed.

Marian continues, "A relative and I were visiting Alan, and when we arrived, a surgeon was at the desk talking to the nurses. My companion laughed and said, 'Hello, it looks as though someone is scheduled for a chop.' At the time we didn't realize it was Alan. Screens were in place around his bed. The surgeon told me that things weren't good at all and they were going to have to amputate both legs. He said whether they would cut above or below the knee depended on what they found.

"I couldn't take it in," Marian says. "I was in shock. I thought they might only take his toes, because I had seen a form by his bed that said his toes had gangrene. I knew his feet were in a terrible state. But it was clearly more serious than that."

By now, Marian recalls, Alan was very unwell. He was in a lot of pain. His body was burning with fever and he was rambling again. He was glistening with sweat and was covered with red blotches. They later learned that those red patches were hundreds of blood clots located just under his skin. Marian continues, "One of the doctors I had come to know told me it was unlikely Alan would survive. His kidneys had failed, his lungs were close to failing, and his heart was badly affected. When I heard this, I felt like I had to get out of there. I had to get home and speak to our four children. I felt guilty about leaving, but I couldn't stay there any longer.

"I went home and told the children how sick Alan was. The hospital called to say he was on his way to surgery, and then we heard nothing for hours. We all expected the worst; we thought he was going to die. It got to be 6:00 P.M. and my son said he couldn't stand the waiting anymore, so he phoned the hospital. When he got through to Alan's ward, he started shouting that his dad was alive and in intensive care.

"We went to the hospital and my son ran up the stairs while the rest of us waited for the elevator. When we got there, our son was outside the ward and crying. He said that it wasn't his dad in there. Alan was six feet two before the amputation, so in his bed with a cage over his stumps he looked so small. The nurses did move the cage down to make him look a bit better, but it was hard for all of us to see him that way."

Marian says no one knows how many strokes Alan suffered before the operation, but once his legs were amputated, he began to recover. His eyesight was affected and he still rambled, but she could see a positive change in him. She says, "The doctors didn't know what to do with him; they were quite honest about it. One doctor in intensive care came to me and said, 'How do you think he is?' I thought, 'Why ask me? You're the doctor.'

"From the moment Alan's legs were removed from below the knee, his recovery began. His platelet count began to rise and he was started on heparin intravenously. Later, that was changed to warfarin. Even in those first days in intensive care, Alan was obviously getting better. His real improvement came when he was allowed to go home. I could have a conversation with him again. A few months later he had some artificial legs made; that was the middle of July. By Christmas he was walking pretty well with the help of canes. He has never looked back since."

Marian was told that Alan had made medical history by surviving catastrophic antiphospholipid syndrome. At the time, he was the only known patient in the U.K. to have pulled through.

Alan says, "One of the worst things was my eyesight being affected so that I couldn't drive. I had to give up my license. Other than that I now swim regularly at a disabled swimming club, I have a part-time job working from home, and my health is as good as ever. I truly am a lucky man!"

What to Do

If you experience any of the following symptoms, especially if you know that you carry the antiphospholipid antibodies, get yourself to a hospital immediately. If applicable, be sure to tell the nurses and doctors in the ER about your having tested positive for the APLA:[3]

- ◆ If you're pregnant, the signs of miscarriage, including cramping, vaginal bleeding, and vaginal discharge;

- ◆ Extremely low or nonexistent urine production (can indicate a cutoff of blood to the kidneys);

- ◆ Confusion, loss of coordination, loss of consciousness, seizures, loss of vision, unexplained changes in behavior, emotional instability (can indicate a cutoff of blood to the brain);

- ◆ Labored breathing, a nonproductive cough (can indicate a cutoff of blood to the lungs);

- ◆ Acute chest pain, sudden hypertension (can indicate a cutoff of blood to the heart);

- ◆ Abnormally low blood pressure;

◆ Dark-bluish or purple patches on the skin, especially at
  the extremities;

◆ Severe abdominal cramping and pain.

Treatment usually involves a combination of immunosuppressive and anticoagulation drugs, steroids, and plasmapheresis (a
procedure that lowers the amount of plasma in the blood).

Although potentially fatal, CAPS is also extremely rare. And
when treated properly and in time, many CAPS patients can
recover completely.

Chapter 12

Tests and Treatment
for APS

As I have said repeatedly throughout the book, and as our patients' stories bear out, the key to tackling antiphospholipid syndrome is getting a diagnosis. The most fundamental way to achieve this is to undergo the blood tests specifically designed to detect antibodies linked to the illness. If you suspect you have Hughes syndrome, then ask to be tested. The test costs little and will either put your mind at rest or confirm your fears and help you to the next stage, which is getting treatment.

Two blood tests are currently being used for APS, and they are both widely available in major clinics across the world. You don't have to understand the science behind them; what is important is that you remember the names of the tests so you can insist on having them carried out. There are two tests because slight differences exist between them, and some patients may show a positive result on one but not on the other. To eliminate the uncertainty caused by that discrepancy, it is normal to carry out both.

Anticardiolipin Antibodies

This is an inexpensive test and is so common that it has become standardized in many laboratories worldwide. The lab will separate out the blood's serum (watery portion) and place a drop of it on a glass slide that contains protein and phospholipid. The test measures the blood's actual antibody levels. If you are positive, you will be told whether your aCL levels are low, medium, or high. The higher the aCL level, the greater the risk of thrombosis.

Lupus Anticoagulant

The name of this test is misleading: It is not a test for lupus. It was first identified half a century ago and is a complex blood-clotting test. Those who work with APS say the test is less reliable than the one for anticardiolipin antibodies and is more prone to variations between laboratories. But until a replacement test is found, doctors cannot take the risk of avoiding this test in case the results from the test come back positive.

Usually one positive result will not be enough to confirm a diagnosis of Hughes syndrome. Patients are asked to come back after a few weeks and be retested. Although it is rare, one may test positive the first time and negative the second. No one is sure why this happens. To offset this possibility, doctors also look for clinical indications of APS.

Clinical Clues

When you see a specialist who knows about APS, he or she will look beyond blood tests, which can fluctuate between positive and negative. The doctor will also look for physical signs that you have Hughes syndrome. These include the following:

- ◆ painful joints

- ◆ eye problems

- ◆ a medical history of miscarriage

- ◆ blood-clotting

- headaches

- strokes

When the doctor examines you, he or she will also look for the following:

- blotchy skin

- blue to black fingers and toes

Recall from Chapter 2 that one clotting episode, plus positive blood tests for the APLA, is considered definitive for diagnosing APS.

Treatment

There is a simple logic to treating Hughes syndrome: The blood is more viscous than it should be, so the obvious remedy is to thin the blood. One other way of dealing with the condition exists, and that is to try to suppress the antibodies that cause the problems in the first place. However, this is a tricky proposition as it involves interfering with an already abnormal immune system.

Doctors prefer to target the clotting tendency. They prescribe a number of drugs known as *anticoagulants*, which thin the blood. The treatment may sound frightening, but evidence indicates few side effects with this range of medication. Sometimes a patient may bleed heavily, but with the right monitoring that can be dealt with. The benefits of taking these drugs can be substantial; their effectiveness for the APS sufferer can appear within days or, in some cases, hours.

Three anticoagulant drugs are commonly used to treat APS: aspirin, warfarin, and heparin.

Aspirin

The miracle drug of the last century is still working its magic in the new millennium. Aspirin has long been recognized for its ability to make blood platelets less "sticky." Well beyond the field of Hughes syndrome, aspirin is also used to treat those who have thrombosis, heart disease, or strokes. Low-dose aspirin—even in the amounts contained in so-called baby aspirin—is regarded as a brilliant blood thinner, having the fewest side effects. In rare cases a patient may be allergic to aspirin, but if that's a problem, other drugs exist in the pharmaceutical armory that will also do the job with APS.

In milder cases of this condition, taking aspirin shows clear benefits. Some patients who have gotten through a serious episode and are now generally well take only aspirin to control their symptoms. One area where aspirin shows its effectiveness is in pregnancy. In the lupus pregnancy clinic at St. Thomas' Hospital, the administration of aspirin helped dramatically improve the success rate among women who suffered recurrent miscarriage.

Individuals who take aspirin regularly may find it advisable to take coated aspirin, as it is less prone to cause irritation to the stomach lining over the long term.

Heparin

This is perhaps the least popular treatment of the three, as it must be administered by injection, usually subcutaneously (beneath the skin) at the side of the stomach or thigh. Patients can learn how to inject themselves. Doctors tend to avoid using this treatment over a long period of time.

Heparin does have the following advantages:

◆ It is possible to reverse its blood-thinning effects quite quickly, which is useful if a patient needs surgery.

◆ Heparin is safe to use throughout pregnancy, whereas warfarin cannot be used during pregnancy.

◆ Heparin works much more quickly than warfarin; it can take effect within hours, whereas warfarin can take a day or so to kick in.

Warfarin

Warfarin, which is known in some countries by its brand name, Coumadin, is the standard treatment for thrombosis. It is widely prescribed to treat strokes and TIAs (transient ischemic attacks, or mini-strokes). It has been shown to be highly effective in the long-term treatment of Hughes syndrome. It is relatively free of side effects and is taken orally as a pill. Once a patient is on the medication, he or she must undergo regular INR tests (see below) to monitor the thickness of the blood.

The correct dose of warfarin is found by a process of trial and error. The aim is to keep the blood two or three times thinner than it would normally be, depending on the severity of the symptoms.

INR

INR, which stands for *internationally normalized ratio*, is a measurement used to compare the thickness of a patient's blood with that of normal blood. The higher the ratio, or INR, the thinner the blood. Most patients feel well with an INR of between 3 and 4. Some need it to be even thinner and feel best with an INR of 3.5 to 4. In any event, people being treated for Hughes syndrome are required to have their INR tested regularly.

When you first start taking a blood thinner, it may require several weeks of checking and rechecking your INR and adjusting the dosage of your medication before you and your doctor hit upon the best dosage for you. Many APS patients become familiar with the INR range within which they feel their best.

The name of the test for INR is *prothrombin time* (also called *protime*, or *PT*). Most people who need their INR checked on a regular basis must go to a hospital or lab for PT tests, but self-testing machines are available, with which a patient can keep an eye on her or his INR at home. These machines are extremely useful, but unfortunately they are also expensive.

What You Should Know about Blood Thinners and Your INR

People taking anticoagulants on a regular basis should be aware that many things can affect their INR. The following is a partial list of them:

◆ Foods high in vitamin K. Vitamin K is directly involved in the body's clotting reactions, so people taking blood thinners need to be as consistent as possible in their vitamin K intake from day to day. Vitamin K is found in many foods, but a primary source is green, leafy vegetables. Advice from medical professionals says to consume close to the same amount of these foods every single day, but many people who get regularly tested for their INR find it easier to simply avoid foods high in vitamin K altogether

◆ Other changes in diet

◆ Other medications, including antibiotics and, in some cases, the influenza vaccine

◆ Some over-the-counter drugs, including acetaminophen (Tylenol)

◆ Herbal remedies

◆ Other nutritional supplements, including vitamins and minerals

◆ Alcohol intake. Health professionals generally advise against drinking alcohol at all while taking anticoagulants

◆ Travel

If you are regularly taking an anticoagulation drug, keep your doctor advised about any alterations in your diet, prescription medications, over-the-counter drugs, nutritional supplements, travel habits, or other aspects of your lifestyle.

Other Considerations When Taking a Blood Thinner

People on anticoagulants generally bleed and bruise more easily and take longer to heal. That's because their blood takes longer to clot. Excessive bleeding can lead to anemia in the long term and, of course, dangerous levels of blood loss in the short term. For this reason, individuals taking any of these drugs should observe the following precautions:

- A woman's menstrual flow may increase substantially. Excessive loss of menstrual blood is a leading cause of anemia in women. If your menstrual flow seems excessive, talk to your doctor. He or she can recommend several ways of dealing with this problem.

- Be more careful to avoid injury. If you participate in contact sports or other risky recreational activities, you may need to rethink your recreational choices—or at least rethink the level at which you participate.

- Wear medic alert jewelry, or carry a medic alert card in your wallet. Varieties are available that indicate the wearer is on anticoagulants.

- In the event of an injury that causes bleeding that can't be stopped quickly, go immediately to the emergency room. Let the nurses and doctors there know that you're taking an anticoagulant.

- Alert your family members, close friends, and coworkers of the necessity of dealing quickly with any blood loss you experience.

◆ Report to your doctor any bleeding that occurs for no obvious reason, including nosebleeds, bleeding gums, bloody stools, blood in the urine.

Finally, be reminded of the recommendation given in Chapter 4 that you should *always* request a second opinion from a doctor familiar with APS *before* agreeing to be taken off your anticoagulant treatment, even in preparation for surgery or dental work. Hughes syndrome patients who stop taking their anticoagulants for even a short time often stand a chance of suffering a clotting episode.

In Conclusion

APS can be a disheartening and frustrating condition. Yet, as so many patients have attested in these pages, when the illness is properly diagnosed and treated, recovery can seem miraculous. If you suspect or know that you have Hughes syndrome, resolve to do whatever it takes to get the treatment that is right for you. Realize that doing so may require persistence and backbone. Educate yourself about the disease, stand up for yourself when necessary, and, most of all, refuse to give up. Following these words of advice should help you in your quest to live well with antiphospholipid syndrome.

Notes

1. Adapted from Malerman, Newton. *The Prostate Health Workbook.* Alameda, CA: Hunter House, 2002; Nichols, Judith Lynn (Ed.). *Women Living with Multiple Sclerosis.* Alameda, CA: Hunter House, 1999; "Antiphospholipid Antibody Syndrome" (pamphlet), by Kay Thackray and Marvin Nelson. Available through the APLSUK online support group (hosted by Yahoo; see above). Also available from either author via e-mail. Contact them at kaythackary@aol.com or gldpros@aol.com.

2. "Antiphospholipid Antibody Syndrome" (pamphlet), by Kay Thackray and Marvin Nelson. Available through the APLSUK online support group (hosted by Yahoo; see above). Also available from either author via e-mail. Contact them at kaythackary@aol.com or gldpros@aol.com.

3. Article accessed at www.thedoctorwillseeyounow.com/articles/arthritis/caps_9/#2.

Resources

Organizations

The Hughes Syndrome Foundation (U.K.)
The Rayne Institute: St. Thomas' Hospital
London SE1 7EH England   Tel.: +44-20-7960-5561
Fax: +44-20-7633-0462   Website: www.hughes-syndrome.org

The Lupus Trust (U.K.)
The Rayne Institute: St. Thomas' Hospital
London SE1 7EH England   Tel.: +44-20-7922-8197
Fax: +44-20-7960-5698   Website: www.lupus.org.uk
E-mail: Barbara@lupus.org.uk

Lupus Foundation of America
1300 Piccard Dr., Ste. 200
Rockville MD 20850-4303   Tel.: (301) 670-9292
Fax: (301) 670-9486   Website: www.lupus.org

American College of Rheumatology
1800 Century Place, Suite 250
Atlanta GA 30345   Tel.: (404) 633-3777
Fax: (404) 633-1870   Website: www.rheumatology.org
E-mail: acr@rheumatology.org
The website includes a directory of rheumatologists in the U.S., which
may be useful for finding doctors who know about APS.

American Hospitals that Have Shown an Interest in APS

The Antiphospholipid Syndrome Collaborative Registry (APSCORE)
University of North Carolina at Chapel Hill
Tel.:(919) 966-0572
E-mail: apscore@med.unc.edu

This is a national, NIH-funded project that often handles questions from patients and helps people find local physicians with expertise in APS. The following hospitals are listed in the registry because they have one or more physicians that are actively involved in APS patient care (as well as research):

UNC Healthcare, University of North Carolina at Chapel Hill (Chapel Hill, NC)

Hospital for Special Surgery, Weill/Cornell School of Medicine (New York, NY)

Johns Hopkins University Medical Center (Baltimore, MD)

Duke University Medical Center (Durham, NC)

University of Utah (Salt Lake City, UT)

University of Texas Health Science Center at San Antonio (San Antonio, TX)

Morehouse School of Medicine (Atlanta, GA)

Websites

http://groups.yahoo.com/
A search at this site for "APLSUK" will lead you to an excellent online support group with over 230 members. Membership is required to view the message archives and to post messages. Members can also access the bookmarks section, which provides access to many more links. Other, smaller Yahoo-hosted groups related to APS can be found by searching at this site under "antiphospholipid."

http://forums.delphiforums.com/apsantibody/messages
This is another great online support group. Membership is required to post messages, but anyone can view the archived messages.

www.aarda.org
American Autoimmune Related Diseases Association, Inc., offers information on many autoimmune conditions, including APS.

www.healthcyclopedia.com/antiphospholipid_syndrome.html
A page in an online encyclopedia that features several links to articles on APS/Hughes syndrome.

www.stroke.org
Website of the National Stroke Association.

www.strokesurvivors.org
Website of Strokesurvivors International.

www.fertilityplus.org/faq/miscarriage/resources.htm
Fertility Plus is a nonprofit website covering topics about trying to conceive.

www.womens-health.org.uk
Women's Health Information is a site dedicated to women's health. Search under topics such as "recurrent miscarriage" or "antiphospholipid syndrome."

www.migraines.org
Website of the National Migraine Association (also known as M.A.G.N.U.M.). Includes links to a migraine forum and message board.

Further Reading

Hughes Syndrome: A Patient's Guide, by Graham Hughes, M.D. (Springer Publishing; www.springer.de). Also available through the Hughes Syndrome Foundation website.

"Hughes Syndrome Booklet," by Graham Hughes, M.D. Available through the Hughes Syndrome Foundation website.

Sticky Blood Explained, by Kay Thackray, with a foreword by M. A. Khamashta, M.D. (Author Publishing Ltd., 2003). Available through the Hughes Syndrome Foundation website. Also available through www.amazon.co.uk.

"Antiphospholipid Antibody Syndrome" (pamphlet), by Kay Thackray and Marvin Nelson. Available through the APLSUK online support group (hosted by Yahoo; see above). Also available from either author via e-mail. Contact them at kaythackary@aol.com or gldpros@aol.com.

Hughes Syndrome: Antiphospholipid Syndrome, M. A. Khamashta, ed. (Springer Publishing; www.springer.de). A clinical and scientific guide for doctors and researchers, with contributions from fifty-seven of the world's leading authorities. Available through the Hughes Syndrome Foundation website.

Index